From the author of the best selling Tool I

D0571330

THE INSIDER'S
GUIDE TO
THE NHS

How it works and why it sometimes doesn't

Roy Lilley

WITHDRAWN

Radclif

Radcliffe Medical Press Ltd
18 Marcham Road
Abingdon
Oxon OX14 1AA
United Kingdom

www.radcliffe-oxford.com
The Radcliffe Medical Press electronic catalogue and online ordering facility.
Direct sales to anywhere in the world.

British Library Cataloguing in Publication Data

A catalogue record for this book is available from the British Library.

ISBN 1 85775 874 9

Typeset by Joshua Associates Ltd, Oxford
Printed and bound by TJ International Ltd, Padstow, Cornwall

CONTENTS

ABOUT THE AUTHOR

Roy Lilley was formerly a visiting fellow at the Management School, Imperial College London. He is a writer and broadcaster on health and social issues and has published over two dozen books on health and health service management and related topics.

He has been an *insider* in the NHS for around 25 years.

Previously the vice-chair of a Health Authority, in his time as a NHS Trust chairman his organisation became the first to achieve BS 5750 (ISO 9001) quality accreditation for the whole of its services, along with *Investors in People* approval for the whole of its HR and training strategies. The Trust agreed the only 'no-strike' deal in the NHS.

All staff took part in performance management and everyone had a personal development plan.

He was the chairman of the NHS Trusts Federation's national standing committee on supplies and purchasing and, later, the chairman of the national standing committee on human resource issues. He has been a member of national committees on improving opportunities for women working in the NHS and training for non-executives.

Roy Lilley now writes, broadcasts and works across the NHS to help with the challenges of modern management and is an enthusiast for radical policies that address the real needs of patients, professionals and the communities they serve.

DEDICATION

This guide is dedicated to the army of NHS staff who go to work and struggle to find their way through the increasingly labyrinthine service that has more targets than a rifle range and more pilots than easyJet.

And to the battalions of people with ideas, products and services they want to sell to the NHS, but can never find the front door!

GETTING THE BEST FROM THIS BOOK

Beware! This is a book with attitude, not just a guide, handbook or the usual directory. It tells you about the organisations that make up the NHS and gives you a commentary on what they do, how they do it and how they stand. It is an insider's perception – me!

On the way you'll find:

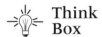 **Think Box**

Think boxes – they are there to get 'the juices flowing' and to get you thinking 'outside the box', to look at the issues and organisations from a different dimension. Some are deliberately provocative, some just for fun.

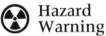 **Hazard Warning**

Hazard warnings, to let you know 'this bit is tricky' or could be a problem.

✓ There are **Tips**, for short-cuts and bright ideas.

. . . and the inevitable ☕, a good place to sit down, make a cup of coffee and have a think!

☺ There are also a few of these. I'm not sure what they mean! I've put them in where there is a comment to make, something I agree with, or a good point – I think!

And, of course, there are the www links to organisations. I've tested them all, at the time of writing, but they do change. So you may have to do a bit of digging. If you get stuck, try entering everything before the first forward slash to take you to the front page, and navigate from there.

INTRODUCTION

This book is aimed at anyone who wants to understand the NHS better.

It is a guide, but not in the sense of a route map or plan. It has useful stuff, such as contact details and web addresses. But if you want a long list of mailing addresses or the names of people who will have moved on by the time you get to read about them – get your money back. This is not the book for you.

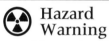

Hazard Warning

Frankly, in this day and age, if you can't do the web stuff you're as good as dead.

To make the information in this book really work you will probably want to get onto the Internet. All the links you need to take you to the boring stuff are here. You can download what you need and turn it into PowerPoint^{TM} slides, lists, executive summaries and all that other stuff that might impress your boss and save your miserable career.

☺ This book has comment, opinion, judgements, views and an attitude. The NHS is struggling under an avalanche of ideas, initiatives, proposals, plans, schemes and ideas – new ideas, daft ideas, stunning ideas, brilliant ideas and the plain stupid ideas. The book aims to take you on the inside track on the component organisations that make up today's fast-changing NHS.

As well as telling you where all this is happening, it encourages you to think about what they are doing and how we will know if they are a success. The idea is: read this book and you will '*know*' about the NHS, be able to debate it, gossip and impress the bloke in the chip shop. The one who thinks he's Elvis. He'll think you are the Secretary of State for Health!

By the way, I know there is a bit of overlap in the book. Some outfits get more than one mention. This is where organisations have natural links with each other, or new organisations are appearing, taking over some or all of the responsibilities of their predecessor.

I hope you find it useful!

Roy Lilley
September 2003

ACUTE TRUSTS

Acute care trusts, bit of an old-fashioned phrase these days. Most people call them 'NHS Trusts' or secondary care. In real life it includes mental health, community and ambulance trusts.

January 2002 will prove to be something of a red letter day in the annals of healthcare history. The Government announced that three star hospitals will have the opportunity to apply to become Foundation Hospitals.

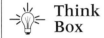 **Think Box**

If Foundation Hospitals are the answer, what is the question?

The attraction is they will have greater power to make their own management and financial decisions with minimal Government intervention.

On the downside, hospitals which persistently underperformed will have their management franchised, meaning they could be run by charities or the private sector as well as the public sector.

TRUSTS IN ENGLAND

There are a couple of ways to become the oracle on English Trusts. First try:

• www.doh.gov.uk/codes/abouto.htm

and then:

• www.doh.gov.uk/codes/datafiles.htm

There is also a list at:

• www.nhs.uk/localnhsservices/list_orgs.asp?ot=R__

☺ In short, there are 271 Trusts, 30 are ambulance trusts, 24 are mental health trusts, 4 community trusts and 213 acute or combined trusts.

Foundation Hospitals really are worth a closer look. They are at the centre of a hearts-and-minds battle for the Government. New Labour and old Labour locked in mortal combat.

Have a look at:

- www.doh.gov.uk/nhsfoundationtrusts/index.htm

Here's a summary of what's on offer for the foundation brigade:

- free from direct management by the Department of Health
- able to make independent decisions on investment
- free to decide how their staff should be paid
- entitled to keep proceeds from land sales to finance new patient services.

If this all sounds a bit like the Thatcher reforms of the early 90s, it is because it's pretty much the same. All of these so-called freedoms are incorporated in the NHS and Community Care Act of 1990.

However, there is a bit of a new spin that has to be added.

- Foundation Hospitals will be not-for-profit organisations 'representing a middle ground between the public and private sector'.

 Think Box

A giant leap forward for public services or a small step towards a two tier system? Whaderyerfink?

- Their assets will be publicly owned but they will be protected from private sector takeovers.
- They will be paid by results, receiving extra resources for taking on more patients.

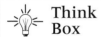 **Think Box**

The Mother-of-All-Battles is about to be commenced. The Gods of Whitehall are very keen and the devils on the back benches are not. The Tories would like to support the idea, as it is based on one of their better ideas from the days when they had policies, ideas and leadership. However, they will oppose Foundation Hospitals on the spurious grounds that the policy 'doesn't go far enough'. The Lib-Dems . . . Well, they say no to most things.

The Department of Health summarises the benefits of foundation status as follows.

- Part of the NHS family, providing healthcare to NHS patients within a framework of national standards but not line managed by the Department of Health.
- Held to account locally by the communities they serve and through 'cash for performance' contracts – based on regulated price tariffs.
- Inspected by CHAI to a set of national standards along with all NHS and independent healthcare providers (for more on CHAI, *see* page 14).
- Provided with new governance structures to reflect the different relationships with patients, staff, the local community and other key stakeholders in order to enhance accountability within the local community.
- Given additional freedoms.
- Established as free-standing legal entities.

Apart from having to have a three star rating, Trusts applying for foundation status will be judged on:

- financial management
- clinical standards
- responsiveness to patients
- leadership and management
- commitment and support from clinical and other staff and local stakeholders.

In other words – everything!

Acute sector bed numbers

We are told that the wizards of modern healthcare and big-pharma have combined to produce minimally invasive treatments and pills instead of operations. So, in theory, we should need fewer beds in the NHS.

Well, the NHS defies gravity, logic and the 10 times table. Apparently we need more beds.

Have a look at:

• www.doh.gov.uk/hospitalactivity

> ✓ The English NHS went from 1971 to 2001 without increasing bed numbers. In September 2001 the number of general and acute hospital beds in the NHS increased by over 700. In fact it was the largest increase since records began in 1960.

This put the Government about one third of the way towards its NHS Plan target of 2100 extra general and acute hospital beds by April 2004.

By 2002 the total increase was 1503.

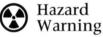 **Hazard Warning**

However, there is more to the numbers than just numbers!

• There were reductions in beds for patients with learning disabilities because institutions have been closed and people are looked after in the community, in their 'own homes', often under the general care of social services.
• A considerable reduction in maternity beds for no reason other than that women are discharged earlier. Whether or not that is a good thing – I dunno!

A WORD ABOUT THE STARS

How are hospital star ratings calculated? Go see:

- www.doh.gov.uk/performanceratings/

The idea is raise the national standards. The best Trusts get three stars and the chief executive gets to keep their job. The worst get no stars. If nothing improves, the chief executive can expect to get the sack. Simple!

The three star-ers have a bit more freedom to manoeuvre. They get control over how they spend money, less inspections and the opportunity to directly advise the Government on NHS policy. Oooh!

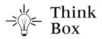 **Think Box**

Do stars and targets work? If you are in the private sector you will have targets, that's for sure. In the NHS, the production line workers, the medics, say targets distort clinical priorities. In other words, they want to make the choices.

Might they be right?

One thing is for certain, talk to any patient and the one thing they worry about the most is having to wait to be treated. All of the focus-group stuff and the opinion surveys put waiting at the top of the worry list.

AUDIT COMMISSION

Forget Google, here it is:

• www.audit-commission.gov.uk/home/

Audit Commission
1 Vincent Square
London SW1P 2PN
Tel: 020 7828 1212

WHAT DOES IT DO?

You pay the taxes and the public sector spends 'em. Where does the money go and is it well spent? Reasonable questions. It was a question thought about by a well known politician, a household name in his day.

Some say the best prime minister we never had.

 This is interesting stuff, but as they are on the way out of healthcare, if you are in a rush, go to the section on CHAI.

None other than Tory politician, now retired, Michael Heseltine. Back in the Thatcher years of Government, Heseltine was a Secretary of State with a difference. A background in the private sector. He had founded and developed Haymarket Publishing into a huge business. It was his business background and 'business-like' thinking that drove him to ask the question: 'Where does the money go and is it well spent?' The result was that he set up the Audit Commission.

A body independent of Government, the Audit Commission is responsible for the three Es: ensuring that public money is used:

• economically
• efficiently
• effectively.

Not just an inspectorate, the Audit Commission conducts research on public sector delivery performance, and:

• participates in joint inspections
• is responsible for best value inspection of public services not covered by other statutory inspectorates

- is also responsible for appointing external auditors to audit the financial statements and to carry out reviews of governance arrangements and performance in all local authorities, health authorities, trusts and local health groups in Wales, police and fire authorities and national parks authorities.

At least, it did!

CHAI

> ✓ There are some changes that will be made.

In 2002 the Secretary of State for Health decided he wanted a bit more specialised inspection and set up the Commission for Healthcare Audit and Inspection (*see* page 14).

This will carve out the Audit Commission's role in healthcare and roll it up with the work of the Commission for Health Improvement and the National Care Standards Commission (NCSC), *who were supposed to be inspecting the healthcare provided by the private sector*. Private sector?

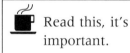 Read this, it's important.

Is that important?

Yes, the Government has made it clear it doesn't care where the healthcare is delivered from, public or private sector. Therefore inspections, standards and guidelines become more important to ensure consistency across a mixed economy of suppliers.

Here's what CHAI will do.

- Everything that CHI used to do plus the stuff in the NHS Reform and Healthcare Professions Act (2002), *don't worry about the details of that*.
- Everything that the NCSC was going to do in the private sector.
- All the value-for-money stuff the Audit Commission did – and they aren't too pleased to be relieved of the job. Expect a bit of a turf war!

CHAI will be busy, they have to:

- report on all NHS hospitals once a year
- make recommendations for special measures where there are persistent problems, foul-ups and failures

- license private healthcare provision
- figure out if healthcare is giving value for money – that's the old job pinched from the Audit Commission

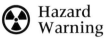 **Hazard Warning**

See, it's the private sector again. There will be a blurring of the boundaries between what's public and what's private. No one cares if it's public or private, providing it's good enough. Well, no one except a tidy number of Labour's backbench politicians.

- when they know how well the NHS is doing, they will publish reports and carry on with the barmy idea of star-rating hospitals – although gossip has it that star ratings may be dropped.

. . . and, as if to prove they are independent of politicians and political string-pulling, they will publish an annual report to Parliament, covering such things as how well the money is being spent, whether it is value for money and what progress the NHS is making.

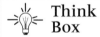 **Think Box**

Question: if the NHS gets a bad report, what happens then? Who eats the carrots and who gets hit with the sticks? When you find out, give me a ring and let me know!

Remember, CHAI is supposed to be independent of Government and the NHS. It is the health equivalent of OFSTED for schools. We could call CHAI OFFSICK, but they don't like it!

There is a big question over CHAI's ability to deliver. Not because they are idiots; they are not. It is because of the size of the task. They will have to report on close-on 3000 NHS and NHS supplier establishments every year. If they are to do it with the present approach – inspections – it seems to me one half of the NHS will have to close down whilst it inspects the other half!

In fact, the legislation says CHAI must report on each establishment every year and 'may inspect'. So, there is a let-out. CHAI's boss and executive chairman (the only one in the NHS), Professor Sir Ian Kennedy (yes, it's him, the Kennedy Report into the Bristol baby scandal), says he wants to work by 'holding a mirror up to the NHS'. Nice phrase that. I like it. What does it mean? I'm not sure! I think it means he wants Trusts to be able to compare performance based on data and what-not. That sounds good to me. The trouble is the NHS is about 10 years away from being able to do it.

In the meantime, what happens? Dunno! I think CHAI's reports might come under pressure from an already sceptical press.

Watch this space . . .

 CHAI is a very important organisation and there is more about them on page 14. It is a must-read, really.

CARE TRUSTS

For an in-depth explanation try:

☢	**Hazard Warning**

Already an endangered species?

• www.doh.gov.uk/caretrusts/

There aren't too many Care Trusts about. At the time of writing there are only a handful:

• Bradford District Care Trust
• Camden and Islington Mental Health and Social Care Trust (www.cimhscaretrust.nhs.uk/)
• Manchester Mental Health and Social Care Trust
• Northumberland (www.northumberlandcaretrust.nhs.uk/), which came via the PCT route
• Witham, Braintree & Halstead, the last remaining PCG, became a Care Trust in October 2002.

Two Care Trusts providing mental health services were launched in April 2003, they are:

• Sheffield
• Sandwell.

What are they?

Care Trusts do the obvious. They care! Don't all Trusts? Yes, but these are special, they care for some very vulnerable people.

They merge together health and social services into one organisation. Some would say this is a long overdue initiative and the whole of the NHS should do it. However, Care Trusts are run by health and not social services.

That means local government, previously responsible for social services, lose part of their empire. Most of them are not too keen on the idea, hence the uptake of Care Trusts has been slower than the gods of Whitehall might have liked, in providing 'seamless delivery' of care and thereby breaking down the barriers that have existed between the two services. However, because the new bodies will be NHS-controlled, local authorities are concerned that this will give the NHS control over the service previously supplied by them.

For the most part Care Trusts focus on the needs of people with mental health problems and the elderly, the two groups of service users who have a high dependency on social services and struggle with the artificial boundaries that exist between the two services.

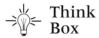 **Think Box**

In a patient-focused environment you might think there would be more Care Trusts?

What's the problem?

In short, the NHS is free at the point of need and some social services are means tested. See the point? Critics are saying that Care Trusts are a short step away from the NHS starting to charge for its services.

☺ Prediction for the future? Care Trusts are too difficult and will wither on the vine.

CHAI

THE COMMISSION FOR HEALTHCARE AUDIT AND INSPECTION

Not much on the website yet. Not really worth a visit.

• www.doh.gov.uk/statementofpurpose/index.htm

Oh what fun this lot is. It's already in a mess! CHAI is the successor organisation to CHI. The new full-time executive chairman is Sir Ian Kennedy (he of the Kennedy Report into the Bristol fiasco fame). It is the first time the NHS has had an executive chairman. The present chief executive of the outgoing CHI, Peter Homa, was earmarked as the new CEO of CHAI.

However, a month or two into the planning stage of CHAI, Kennedy had a row with Homa and Homa stood down.

 Think Box

Everyone in the NHS knows Peter Homa is the world's nicest man, a great manager and trusted! Kennedy must be a tough customer.

Homa made the concept of the predecessor organisation, CHI, acceptable to the NHS because he emphasised the developmental nature of the work, involved people and made it as non-threatening as possible. He even persuaded NHS managers, doctors and nurses that inspecting each other wasn't career-threatening. He did a good job!

Ministers are rumoured to want a tougher inspection regime (CHAI will be inspecting the private sector, too) and, apparently, the row came down to touchy-feely versus boot-in-the-backside. The truth is, we'll never know precisely what the row was about. Homa has kept his mouth shut and Kennedy is keeping his head down.

Watch this space! If CHAI is to be tough then my guess is Kennedy will find it hard to recruit assessors/inspectors from the NHS. They know that putting the boot in on colleagues can be fun at the time but career-threatening a few years later when your victim is sitting on an interview panel!

 Anyway, that's the gossip out of the way. Now, what will it do?

CHI will bring together the Audit Commission, the Commission for Health Improvement and the private healthcare role of the National Care Standards Commission.

It has the job of:

- reporting on all English and Welsh NHS hospitals and cross-border Scottish ones (once a year), with the ability to recommend special measures where there are persistent problems – *this is a huge job, there's a lot of them!*
- licensing private healthcare provision – *previously done by the defunct Care Standards people*
- assessing the value for money of healthcare provision – *previously done by the Audit Commission*

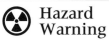

> **Hazard Warning**
>
> This inspection malarkey is such a big job, I have visions of half the NHS closing down, whilst it goes off and inspects the other half!

- publishing reports on the performance of NHS organisations, including 'star ratings' – *the 'old CHI' did this*
- publishing an annual report to Parliament on the progress of healthcare delivery and the use of resources – *new job, helping ministers to distance themselves from the day-to-day running of the NHS.*

Note: A second body, the Commission for Social Care Inspection (CSCI), will bring together the remaining work of the National Care Standards Commission and the Social Services Inspectorate.

COMMUNITY HEALTH COUNCILS

WHERE TO FIND THEM - YOU'LL HAVE TO HURRY

Association of Community Health Councils for England and Wales (ACHCEW)
Earlsmead House
30 Drayton Park
London N5 1PB

THEY ARE ON THE WAY OUT . . .

The idea of a Community Health Council (CHC) goes back to the mid-1970s. They were put in place as patient advocates and to help service users complain. As a watchdog they did a great job.

The NHS Reform and Health Care Professions Bill in June 2002 was their death sentence.

> ☺ If they are on the way out, why waste time on them? Because they are at the centre of a controversy and their successor organisation is important and you need the background.

If you want the CHC's part of the story go to:

- www.achcew.org.uk/PPI%20Briefing.htm

CHCs are being replaced by Patients' Forums. Setting aside this fact and the fact that the CHCs now have an axe to grind, there are some real concerns about how independent the new arrangements will be and whether they will be adequate in terms of resources and experience to do the job?

> ✓ Every year roughly 30,000 people complain about the NHS through their local CHC.

DEPARTMENT OF HEALTH

Where to find them:

Department of Health
Richmond House
Whitehall
London SW1

. . . right opposite Downing Street, near the Cenotaph.
  And at:

* www.doh.gov.uk/about/index.htm

The boss is the Secretary of State for Health, who is responsible to Parliament for:

* everything the Department does!

and particularly:

* finance and the deployment of resources
* the tangle and political minefield of the Private Finance Initiative
* so-called 'strategic communications' – in other words, 'spin'.

There is also a team of ministers and their portfolios of responsibility are divided up as follows:

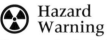 **Hazard**
Warning

I've not included the names of the ministers because they come and go and suddenly decide to spend more time with their families. Great for the kids but it screws up the book publishers!

MINISTER OF STATE FOR HEALTH 1

Responsible for the NHS and delivery of services, including:

* staff and HR functions
* waiting times and access issues

- commissioning
- the use of capital
- primary care services
- health services for asylum seekers
- . . . equality – whatever that means!

MINISTER OF STATE FOR HEALTH 2

Primarily responsible for social care, long-term care, disability and mental health, plus:

- long-term care for the elderly, nursing and residential care
- the new whizzy idea of Intermediate Care
- the social care of children
- General Personal Social Services
- Mental Health Services
- Care Trusts
- health services in prison (generally regarded as a mess)
- long-term conditions, such as diabetes
- renal services and
- services for people with disabilities.

PARLIAMENTARY UNDER SECRETARY OF STATE 1

Broadly, responsible for performance and quality and:

- clinical quality
- pharmaceutical products, medicines and medical devices
- the minefield of genetics and the mysteries of biotechnology
- R&D
- statistics
- the newly refreshed and funded IT agenda
- something called Executive Agency Management – no one has any idea what that's all about
- the day to day management of the Department of Health.

Parliamentary Under Secretary of State for Public Health

This is interesting. Since the formation of the NHS back in 1948 there has never been a minister for public health. It makes sense to have one, as about one third of patients turning up in primary care do so with lifestyle-related illnesses. Labour in its first term of office made a big song and dance about the idea of a public health minister.

Sad to report, very little seems to have been achieved. Poverty, lifestyle and a host of social issues contribute to our health and well-being – or the lack of it. Working across organisational and governmental boundaries to try and address this huge challenge is too much for a junior minister and the opportunity appears lost.

However, this what they are supposed to be doing:

- public health protection and prevention – a huge job when you come to think about it
- cancer
- CHD and stroke
- tobacco, not smoking it – very little real progress
- health inequalities
- embryology – a minefield!
- maternity issues – finding more midwives is no easy task
- SureStart
- children's health
- sexual health and HIV, AIDS
- blood supplies
- teenage pregnancy – try giving away free condoms to the under-16s and see what happens!
- international health business
- Food Standards Agency
- BSE and vCJD
- complementary and alternative medicine – increasing public interest.

Parliamentary Under Secretary of State 2

Bit of a lightweight agenda here, but a good place for a politician to have a go at managing something!

- primarily emergency care
- public involvement – increasingly the sexy buzzword in Government circles
- winter services management
- NHS Direct – with a 98% approval rating from the public but the BMA continue to denounce it
- patients focus – whatever that means
- complaints – plenty of them to keep the minister occupied
- organ retention – oh, a real hot topic
- hospital environment – this means clean, safe places for people to use; not really rocket science but apparently beyond the reach at the moment
- Health Action Zones – a good idea that seems to have fizzled out
- pharmacy services – community pharmacies are under threat from the big multiples
- optical services
- dental services – has anyone seen an NHS dentist recently?
- fluoridation
- drugs, alcohol and its impact on crime
- reconfiguration policy – this is muddled and seems to fit better in another minister's little red box
- occupational health
- appointments – this is really an IT issue – or will be
- Road Traffic Act and charging policy for Trusts
- Defence Medical Services – a confusing cross over with the Department of Defence.

THE ROLE OF THE DEPARTMENT OF HEALTH IS CHANGING

 Think Box

Ministers have realised they can't run the world's largest remaining bureaucracy from a desk in Whitehall. So, they are setting frameworks, targets and guidelines for the service and then inspecting them to see if they've done the job. Makes sense? What do you think? You're paying for it!

Here's what they say they want to achieve:

- set the standards and broad working practices of the NHS and local social services
- monitor how these standards are being met at local level
- take action when they are poor or failing.

Oh, and:

- work on ways to prevent disease and help people live longer, healthier lives – who wouldn't agree with that!

All very nice motherhood-and-apple-pie thinking. Reassuring, don't you think?

The Department of Health is arranged into three main sections:

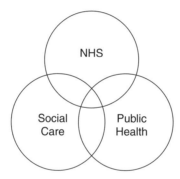

The civil servants who work in the Department are arranged as follows:

- The permanent secretary of the Department of Health, who is also the NHS chief executive. These two roles have recently been combined. He reports to the Secretary of State for Health.

The Department's management board comprises 12 directorates:

- *The strategy unit:* They:
  - develop medium and long-term strategies
  - support the Secretary of State and ministers – I don't think it means taking them home when they've had a few drinks, I think it means helping them think – if you know what I mean!
  - work across departments and Government on strategy
  - bring in external perspectives on strategy and policy.

- *Chief Operating Officer:* He does:
  - NHS performance management
  - access
  - emergency and unscheduled care
  - winter planning
  - acute hospitals
  - liaison with the private sector
  - countering fraud.
- *Children, older people and social care services:* This group look after:
  - health and social care for older people
  - health and social care for children
  - health services for women
  - maternity services
  - general social care policy.

    Plus the Social Services Inspectorate, whose job it is to advise and assist ministers with doing their job around personal social services. They also exercise statutory powers on behalf of the Secretary of State for Health and carry out inspections and performance management.
- *Public involvement, nursing, mental health, disability and allied health professions:* This is a wide-ranging department with responsibility for:
  - patient, user and public involvement
  - nursing, midwifery and health visiting policy
  - mental health policy, services and legislation
  - health and social care policy for people with disabilities and those with long-term conditions
  - allied health professions policy. (They used to be known as PAMs – professions allied to medicine – but for some reason they changed their title. It is people such as physiotherapists and radiographers.)
- *Policy directorate:* Important stuff goes on here. They do:
  - Department of Health policy management, strategy and quality assurance
  - primary care, systems and partnership
  - cancer and heart disease – that's because of all the targets and promises the Government have made about these two disease areas
  - specialist health services, including diabetes, renal and transplant services
  - prison healthcare – there it is again, everyone seems to have prisons on their list, but the services don't get any better!
- *External and corporate affairs:* This looks like a bit of a catch-all department, but interesting none the less. Their responsibilities are:
  - private office

- Department of Health information services
- Department of Health modernisation programme
- equality strategy
- medicines, pharmaceutical and industry issues
- senior appointments and career planning.
- *Communications:* This is what they do:
  - media relations – spin!
  - corporate communications
  - campaigns
  - Public Enquiry Office – have you ever tried using it?

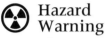 **Hazard Warning**

Given the very poor press the NHS gets it is hard to believe there is a communications department. It must drive ministers barmy.

- *The Modernisation Agency:* This is what they do. There's a lot riding on their being successful:

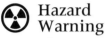 **Hazard Warning**

I must say, I have serious doubts about this . . .

   Modernisation should be everyone's business, not the business of a department or agency. The moment you tribalise it, it becomes some-body else's job. In fairness, the Agency do understand this and try to be as inclusive as possible, but it's a struggle.

- service modernisation
- national clinical governance support team
- national primary care development team
- good practice
- national patients access team
- performance improvement
- modernising the workforce
- changing workforce programme (they do this jointly with the human resources directorate, so they can blame each other if it all goes wrong)
- Leadership Centre
- University of the NHS.
- *Finance:* No prizes for what they do here. However, they have had to buy a bigger bean counter because the Government have given them a whole lot more beans to count:

> ☺ In five years, as a percentage of GDP, NHS funding is going from 7.5% to 9.4%.

- resource planning, acquisition and allocation
- financial management and accounting
- private finance
- capital.
- *Research, analysis and information:* A dark horse department, this one. The aim of this book is not to introduce you to the personalities that work in the NHS (because they change all the time), the aim is to be a quick reference source to what is where. However, it is not possible to describe the work of this group without mention of the man who is in charge. It is Sir John Pattison, a wily Whitehall mandarin who knows every nook and cranny of Government. If there is a task floating around that is in everyone else's 'too difficult tray', it goes into Pattison's tray and gets fixed. However, he will only admit to his top-line functions, which are:
  - economics and operational research
  - statistics
  - research and development
  - information policy
  - genetics.
- *Human resources:* This used to be the personnel department – but the NHS loves the buzzy phrases. Actually, this is a tough brief. The whole of the NHS modernisation agenda really depends on getting more doctors and nurses. It is an uphill struggle.
  A tough job, including:
  - NHS workforce strategy
  - all NHS employment issues
  - workforce planning and development
  - recruitment and retention
  - NHS pay and contracts
  - education
  - training and development for NHS staff
  - regulation
  - changing workforce programme – they do this jointly with the Modernisation Agency, so they can blame each other if it goes wrong!
- *Public health and clinical quality:* This is the preserve of the Chief Medical Officer and includes:
  - public health
  - health protection

- developments and trends in medicine
- incidents and inquiries – this seems to be taking up more and more time
- clinical governance and quality
- patient safety.

SORRY, THERE'S STILL MORE TO COME!

The Department of Health works with five so-called executive agencies. They have what is called 'discrete responsibility' for particular areas. They are still part of the Department and they are:

- *Medical Devices Agency:* looking after the safety, quality and performance of medical devices
- *Medicines Control Agency:* ensuring all medicines on the UK market meet appropriate standards of safety, quality and performance
- *NHS Estates:* responsible for buildings and facilities
- *NHS Pensions Agency:* obvious, no explanation required?
- *NHS Purchasing and Supply Agency:* providing all the kit and caboodle the NHS needs.

Other big cheeses in the Department of Health:

- the Chief Medical Officer (CMO) – the Government's most senior medical advisor
- the Chief Social Services Inspector (CSSI)
- the Chief Nursing Officer – provides advice on nursing, midwifery and health visiting
- the Chief Dental Officer
- the Chief Pharmaceutical Officer for England.

If you want to know more, have a look at:

- www.doh.gov.uk/about/keyspecialists.htm

OK, SO WE KNOW IT'S BIG AND IT'S BEAUTIFUL, BUT WHAT IS IT TRYING TO ACHIEVE?

Always in the headlines, the NHS is undergoing great changes: structural changes, workforce changes and changes in the way it thinks of its customers – the patients.

☺ This is big stuff for the world's largest and oldest nationalised industry to get to grips with. It is a step change in thinking and has the effect of turning the NHS on its head.

Underpinning the change are a number of important documents and guidance changing the direction of travel. Let's look at the most important ones.

For an in-depth look go to:

• www.doh.gov.uk/dhreview/index.htm

In the spring of 2001 the DoH published a paper setting out the future 'shape and direction' of the NHS. Here's a summary of what is in the document.

• Improvements in services and health can only be delivered by the people working directly with patients, clients and the public at the front line. The Department's central focus is to support them in delivery.
• We have to change from a Department that is focused on policy to one that is focused on delivery.

This is how the DoH said it would make the objectives happen:

> To support delivery at the front line we will have clear priorities – and stick to them. The areas where we need to see the biggest improvements are:
> • the conditions with the greatest clinical priority – cancer and coronary heart disease, services for older people and mental health
> • primary care – the point of contact most people have with the NHS
> • emergency care – the services people need to know are there for them when they require them
> • cutting waiting times
> • get the fundamentals of care right, that means looking after people in the right environment and in the right way.
> We will also strengthen local, community and staff ownership of modernisation plans.

✓ Other documents dealing with the 'modernisation' agenda are:
- *The NHS Plan*
- *Modernising Social Services*
- *Our Healthier Nation.*

All of this, the DoH claims, puts the patient, the client and the public at the centre.

An extravagant claim? Well, time will tell. But all the documents and plans were developed through public and stakeholder consultation and involvement in task forces and action teams. This was an unprecedented exercise in consultation.

At the start, as with any round of major changes, the implementation was 'top-down' and drew a good deal of comment from critics who said the approach was too top-heavy. However, the second phase was, in the words of the DoH, intended to be bottom-up, with the emphasis on local ownership.

The DoH summary looks like this:

- Local Modernisation Reviews, to create local three-year implementation plans based on local circumstances and capabilities
- maintaining existing task forces and Modernisation Boards and Councils nationally and regionally, involving stakeholders in policy making and implementation wherever possible
- strengthening partnership with the professions and staff around shared aims and activities (the DoH published a joint statement with the medics and the NHS entitled *A Commitment to Quality, a Quest for Excellence* – heady stuff, eh?)
- supporting a systematic communications programme to ensure local engagement in planning for delivery
- regular meetings and networks of clinicians and managers, involving ministers and the Department's senior staff with patients, clients, the public and staff groups
- improving and simplifying planning processes in the NHS and in local authorities – with the aim of reducing duplication of effort, ensuring consistency and aligning timetables, and supporting integrated working across health services, social care and public health
- decentralising to the most local level.

This is a tall order, but the DoH says it will achieve its task by:

- supporting the development of local and more specialist managed networks based around clinical teams
- developing Primary Care Trusts and giving them maximum control over resources
- creating Strategic Health Authorities – for performance management
- removing the Department's own intermediate tier, so as to create a single system of national performance management and planning
- encouraging local partnerships in health and local government to ensure integrated health and social care services
- focusing on supporting performance improvement at the front line.

Do you see the pattern that is emerging? This is little more than a project management approach. The next step is:

- creating a strong national framework of standards through National Service Frameworks, the National Institute for Clinical Excellence and other means
- providing development support through the Modernisation Agency
- the Social Care Institute of Excellence
- the Leadership Centre
- the University of the NHS and . . .
- developing a unified performance management system within the NHS.

Oh, yes! Where would we be without a bit of the old performance management! The Departmental Change Programme *(sounds like the telly programme 'Changing Rooms', but for ministers . . .)*.

They want to know if they are (their words, not mine) 'adding real value'. How will we know? There's more of this gobbledegook. They say they want to have 'the right people in the right place to lead and deliver change'.

So, they're gonna:

- establish new arrangements for developing leadership, managing senior appointments and career planning in the NHS and the Department
- develop a more systematic approach to managing interchange and shared training between the Department, the NHS, local government, the voluntary and private sectors and other Government departments

- develop greater flexibility and staff development within the Department, including the creation of a pool of staff to respond to emerging issues, a richer skill mix and a new training and development strategy
- improve the working lives of our staff.

. . . Groan . . . Who writes this stuff?

There's loads more, but if you haven't got the idea by now, give up.

For the unreconstructed bobble hat wearer, try the *Department of Health Report 2003–4*. You'll find it at:

- www.doh.gov.uk/dohreport/index.html

Now go and get a life!

WALK-IN CENTRES

Here's the source for the official line:

- www.doh.gov.uk/nhswalkincentres/info.htm

> ☺ This is big sexy stuff. Walk-in Centres were launched by none other than the Prime Minister himself, on the inauspicious 13 April 1999. When he gets involved it's either going to war, or a new initiative on the way. This is a very new initiative that got the NHS very excited – love and hate in equal measure.

Walk-in Centres are 'nurse-led' facilities where you can drop in, without an appointment, and get your minor bits and pieces fixed up.
The official line is:

- Centres must be managed by an NHS body or a GP Co-operative.
- Centres must have support from and/or the endorsement of the local Primary Care Group/Trust, Health Authority, GP Co-operative and the wider local health economy.
- Centres are expected to provide a range of high quality minor ailment and treatment services (and possibly medical minor injuries services) to all patients.
- Centres are expected to provide information about NHS, social services and other local statutory and voluntary services as well as advice about self-care and information and advice about healthy lifestyles, e.g. smoking, diet etc.
- Centres should be in a demonstrably convenient location to enable easy access by the target population – e.g. town centre, adjacent to Accident and Emergency Departments.

> 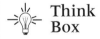 **Think Box**
>
> If these new-fangled places are to be plonked down next to a hospital, why not just have the patient walk in to the hospital?

- Centres should have a responsive style of service (including opening hours which meet patient needs – e.g. early mornings, later evening access and open at weekends).

• Walk-in, immediate access service.

 Think Box

OK, so what is a minor ailment – might seem minor to them, but it's always major to me!

Here's what you've got to have to qualify for this dazzling new service:

• coughs, colds and flu-like symptoms
• minor cuts and wounds – care, dressings
• skin complaints – rashes, sunburn, head-lice, nappy rash
• muscle and joint injuries – strains and sprains
• stomach ache, indigestion, constipation, vomiting and diarrhoea
• women's health problems, e.g. thrush, menstrual advice
• hay-fever, bites and stings
• need information on staying healthy/local services.

Seems to me you could sort most of that lot out with a trip to the chemist! Patients can find their nearest Walk-in Centre by www-ing their way to this website: www.nhs.uk/localnhsservices/wicentres/default.asp.

 Just as this guide was going to press the big policy brains of Whitehall announced £40 million for 10 new Walk-in Centres in London. Good news? Well, the BMA (as usual) had something to say. They were worried that the announcement did not include the money for running the new centres and thought that Primary Care Organisations might pinch the cash from GPs' primary care budgets. And – 10 centres at a cost of four million quid each? Does that sound like a lot of money to you? Either they are as big as Heathrow's new terminal five, or they have gold door-knobs.

HEALTH DEVELOPMENT AGENCY

- www.hda-online.org.uk/

The Health Development Agency was created to improve your health. Feel better for that? No, I thought not!

Anyway, it's probably not interested in you. It's all about reducing health inequalities and improving people's lives.

It aims to do three things:

- find out what works to improve health and create a research and evidence base
- set some standards for practice in public health
- sort out public health strategy and develop the public health workforce.

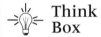

Think Box

The public health profession has been something of a Cinderella job. The truth is, good public health policy is at the heart of reducing demand in healthcare. However, bonny bouncing babies, granny's new hip and whizzo technology make better news for the spin doctors than the back-room work of the real doctors in public health.

The HDA has been going since April 2000 and has somehow accumulated a staff of 120 and a budget of 10 million quid – don't ask how they spend it!

So far it has published 46 papers on public health evidence and best-practice guidelines, including work on stuff like the National Service Framework (NSF), coronary heart disease, the NSF for older people and smoking cessation.

It has also had a delve into the sexual health of young people. To find out what else it's done you can download its annual report from:

- www.hda-online.org.uk/html/about/index.html

PRODIGY

Find them at:

PRODIGY National Dissemination Office (NDO)
Sowerby Centre for Health Informatics at Newcastle (SCHIN)
University of Newcastle
16/17 Framlington Place
Newcastle upon Tyne

Find the full facts by going to:

* www.prodigy.nhs.uk/

. . . and looking for 'Prodigy Guide'.

> ☺ In the dictionary a 'prodigy' is described as a talented and precocious child, or a person endowed with exceptional gifts. In the world of the NHS 'prodigy' means something else.

However, if you can't be bothered – read on.

Prodigy was, a few years ago, another name for a bit of a punch-up. In simple terms, Prodigy is a computer-based system that helps doctors – mainly GPs – to chose the right prescription. It has a nice comfy name; it's called 'decision support'.

However, trust the NHS to make a dog's breakfast of everything. The docs weren't too keen on using Prodigy because they don't like being told what to do – do any of us? The docs thought Prodigy was intrusive and nibbled away at their clinical freedoms. Well, the emotional ones did!

The smart ones realised that Prodigy, as well as giving advice, recorded what the docs actually did. So their performance was capable of being audited. Ouch, they don't like that at all. Well, a lot of them don't.

However, we seem to have moved on. Most GPs have come to realise that Prodigy has a wealth of information that can help them in their daily work. There is no doubt there is a mountain of information that avalanches onto the desks of GPs, and keeping up to date is a nightmare. Prodigy helps with that problem by getting a lot of it on computer so that the inquisitive doc can search and find truth, enlightenment, glory and a few facts.

Now Prodigy is very much part of the day-to-day NHS, accepted and relied upon. Some of the pharmaceutical companies have the odd bitch about the things that Prodigy has to say about their pills, but by and large Prodigy is part of the bricks and mortar of the NHS.

☺ There was a time when it was envisaged that all Prodigy material would be supplied by the National Institute for Clinical Excellence (NICE). However, that got parked in the 'too difficult' tray, and Prodigy picks up its info from many sources.

Envisaged as a step into the happy land of computing, technology and all things whizzy, Prodigy say they are soon to produce their advice in a book! A book? A book? No, I don't understand it either.

 Take a break!

PHARMACEUTICAL INDUSTRY, MEDICINES, PILLS AND POTIONS

 Make a cup of coffee, start at the web address below and be prepared to fall asleep after the first five hours' reading!

* www.doh.gov.uk/medicines.htm

When finished you will know all about the delights of:

* Prepayment, Maternity and Medical Exemptions: FP92/96 statistical returns
* Provision of patient information with dispensed medicines: guidance note
* NHS repeat dispensing schemes in England
* Gluten Free Foods – Local Options (*Oh yes, it's all there!*)
* Pharmacy Workforce in the New NHS, how to make the best use of staff to deliver the NHS Pharmacy Programme
* Prescription Charges: New Arrangements for Issuing Certificates
* Glucosamine/Nutriprem Consultation March–May 2002 – something for the hard-core NHS anoraks
* Measures to control the price of generic medicines sold to community pharmacies and dispensing doctors
* The Pharmaceutical Price Regulation Scheme
* Pharmaceutical Industry Competitive Task Force – Final Report March 2001 (*a sort of 'love-in' between big-pharma and the NHS*)
* Pharmaceutical Industry Competitiveness Task Force – Terms Of Reference
* Ensuring Best Practice in the Notification of Product Discontinuations – Best Practice Guidelines – May 2001
* Local Pharmaceutical Services – *remember them?*

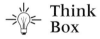 **Think Box**

There's loads more of this technical stuff. It may be just what you're looking for or it may be the sort of stuff that sends you off in a trance.

The bottom line is this; there is a strange relationship between big-pharma and the NHS. Here are some of the issues.

* Pharma makes squillions of pounds, euros and dollars in overseas earnings and the UK treasury loves it.

- Pharma gets tax breaks on R&D, marketing costs and guaranteed earning thresholds, so its results come from an un-level playing field.

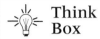 **Think Box**

Who is pharma's customer? Her Majesty's Government, the Department of Health, the doctor prescribing the product or the patient who uses the stuff?

- Pharma employs loads of people but R&D and manufacturing is increasingly being done by computers and robots and clever stuff and the people content is reducing.
- Pharma is running out of what they call 'pipeline' – that is, the next wonder drug that makes them mega-bucks. To conceal their poor performance they keep merging, hiding the real problem of inefficiency.
- Pharma puts millions into R&D, but actually, in real terms, spends more money on marketing than it does on research.
- Pharma's sponsoring department in Government is the Department of Health, its customer, not the Department of Trade and Industry.
- Price controls across the UK and Europe discourage pharma from launching new medicines here and generally it launches first in the US, where it can get its price.
- NHS postgraduate education is, one way and another, almost entirely funded by big-pharma money.
- As more and more of the control of the NHS economy is in the control of Primary Care Organisations, who use formularies, formulary directors and formulary managers, individual doctors have less of a say in what they will prescribe. Pharma field forces and sales staff are becoming less effective. Access to key decision-makers is becoming a real problem.

Get the picture? You either think big-pharma is soft, inefficient, led by fat cats, subsidised and facing a really tough future, or you think big-pharma is a pivotal contributor to the UK economy and a valuable partner in healthcare, without whom continuing professional development for doctors would fall over.

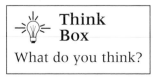
Think Box
What do you think?

Just in case you do wear a bobble hat and collect train numbers, here is some more of the stuff to drool over, to be found at the web address given above:

- Prescription Charges in the UK: Guide for Dispensing Contractors – April 2001
- PCG/PCT Prescribing and Budget-Setting 2001/2
- Prescription
- 2001 Prescription Forms and other information
- Prescription Charges: April 2002 Changes
- Exemption – Guides for Pharmacists and Prescribing Doctors & Electronic Transmission of Prescriptions
- Wider Availability of Emergency Contraception
- NICE Guidance on the Use of Zanamivir (Relenza): Implementation Guidance for NHS – *remember the fuss over this?*
- Local Pharmacy Budgets (indicative) – Domiciliary Oxygen Therapy Services
- Local Pharmacy Budgets 2002/2003 (final) – Domiciliary Oxygen Therapy Services
- Current Consultations
- Completed Consultations
- Consultation on Proposals to Extend Nurse Prescribing, Closed 10 January 2001 – *actually, very important stuff*
- Proposals for Supplementary Prescribing by Nurses and Pharmacists and Proposed Amendments to the Prescription Only Medicines (Human Use) Order 1997
- Consultation on the current Statutory Framework for the Treatment of Impotence on the National Health Service by GPs, 5 February 2001. Last updated: 10/03/2003.

If you are still alive after all that *(check your pulse and see if it is moving)*, there is some more good stuff about the management of medicines at the Audit Commission's website, to be found at:

- www.audit-commission.gov.uk/reports

MEDICINES CONTROL AGENCY

Ooooh, very important people. They live at:

- www.mca.gov.uk

The MCA are there to make sure the pills and potions we take, in the words of the Medicines Act 1968, 'meet appropriate standards of safety, quality and efficacy'. Efficacy – good word, eh?

> ✓ Be sure to get a grip of this.
> The Medicines Control Agency and the Medical Devices Agency (MDA) were merged into a single executive agency from April 2003. The two agencies are accountable for the regulation of medicines and of medical devices.

They are a pretty transparent outfit; they even publish their business plan. You can see it at their website.
   Amongst other tweed-waistcoat stuff there is:

- the Medicines Act *(The whole nine yards, free for download. Read it and drop in the odd comment at the next management meeting and look very impressive)*
- European legislation – the UK's links with Europe are an increasingly important area *(such things as a pan-Europe licensing protocol, the prospect of a pan-Europe NICE)*
- Medicines Commission
- current legal framework
- Committee on Safety of Medicines
- Advisory Board on the Registration of Homeopathic Products *(the public love this stuff and buy it in increasing quantities. Watch out for this sector of the market to keep growing and questions to be raised about more regulation)*
- British Pharmacopoeia Commission
- Independent Review Panel for Advertising.

Oh, yes and

- the Veterinary Products Committee.

Prescription medicines – that means the ones that the doc gives you a prescription for and you then trot off down to the chemist to get – are reimbursed under a very complicated formula that is too horrible to trouble your pretty little head with. However, if you are of the 'two-brains' breed, you might be delighted at:

- www.doh.gov.uk/pprs/index.htm

Ain't technology grand!

And, if you would like to see Whitehall at its creative and obfuscating best, take a look at the masterpiece at:

- www.doh.gov.uk/pictf/index.htm

It's all about the big-pharma industry Competitiveness Task Force.

European Agency for the Evaluation of Medicinal Products (EMEA)

It you are of the anti-Euro persuasion you can throw a brick through their window at:

EMEA
7 Westferry Circus
Canary Wharf
London E14 4HB
UK
Tel: +44 (0)20 7418 8400
Fax: +44 (0)20 7418 8416

☺ You might need a long ladder to do it!

Look, however you feel about Europe, ask yourself this question: 'Are we set for more Euro-stuff, or less?' I think we know the answer.

Codification and standardisation of medicines licensing and control pan-Europe makes sense. Get a medicine licensed in one part of Europe and it is automatically accepted and used in another part – makes sense.

It makes sense for some of the newcomers to Europe who don't have the sophistication of control that some of the 'old Europe' countries take for granted. Pan-European licensing will please the pharma industry who want what they call 'faster access' to markets.

☺ Fast access? In other words, they want to flog the stuff everywhere as soon as it has been licensed. They want to start to get a return on their bucks, and who can blame them?

Avoidance of duplication makes perfect sense, as does a pan-European NICE, to assess the clinical cost-effectiveness of pharma-products.

For the story so far, visit:

• www.emea.eu.int/

You will discover the European system for the authorisation of pharma-stuff started in 1995. Then the European Agency for the Evaluation of Medicinal Products (EMEA) was established by Council Regulation (EEC) No 2309/93 of 22 July 1993. Quote that and look – er, well – dull, boring, a cardigan wearer or a genius! Depends on the company you keep!

Too busy to web-watch? OK, here's what you need to know.

There are two ways to get a pharma-product authorised.

- The so-called 'centralised' procedure. This is a 'must-do' for medicinal products derived from biotechnology and available at the request of pharma-companies for other innovative new products. All the work is done in the UK, at Canary Wharf. They have exactly 210 days to come to a conclusion.
- The decentralised procedure (sometimes called the mutual recognition procedure) is the more usual route. The way it works is called the 'principle of mutual recognition of national authorisations'. In other words, where a product is cleared to be sold in one member state, the others do it too. If there is a problem the EMEA arbitrate. If there is still a problem, the European Commission has the final say.

> ✓ If you are looking for a little stocking filler for Christmas, and you have enough anoraks, pencil sharpeners and Boy Scout badges, you could get hold of a copy of the Review of the European Pharmaceutical Legislation.

There, not too painful, eh?

There is a big-pharma organisation you might just want to know a bit more about. They are the European Federation of Pharmaceutical Industries and Associations (EFPIA) and they live at:

- www.efpia.org/

If you want to pop in and see them, they live at:

Rue du Trône 108
B-1050 Brussels
Belgium

There are some very good restaurants in the neighbourhood, so be sure to take someone with you who has a very big expense account!

If foreign travel in the pursuit of knowledge is outside your reach, you can become an expert on General Pharmaceutical Services in England and Wales at:

- www.doh.gov.uk/public/sb0230.htm

It is a compost heap of richly ripening facts and figures! Stuff such as:

- As of 31 March 2002, 10,463 pharmacies were in contract with health authorities in England and Wales, compared with 10,471 at 31 March 2001, a decrease of 8. *(I wonder what happened to the eight? If you know, write to me!)*
- The percentage of pharmacies in chains of more than 5 rose from 48% in 2000–2001 to 51% in 2001–2002. *(Does this mean the independent trader is on the way out?)*
- In 2001–2002 56% of pharmacies closing were within 500 metres of another pharmacy but 60% of pharmacies opening were more than 1 km from the nearest pharmacy. *(Got that? Just bear in mind some poor soul is sitting somewhere with a map, working all this stuff out!)*

☺ As the great Sir Michael Caine would say, 'Not many people know that!'

I bet you can't wait until the next dinner party to trot out these little show stoppers!

BRITISH NATIONAL FORMULARY (OTHERWISE KNOWN AS THE BNF, OR THE DOC'S BIBLE)

- www.bnf.org/index.htm

This little gem of a book is a joint effort by the Royal Pharmaceutical Society of Great Britain and the docs' trade union, the British Medical Association.

Remember when doctors used to wear white coats? Well this little book is small enough to fit in the pocket of one of those coats. It is a quick reference book designed to:

- be a crib-sheet that helps wise, cost-effective and safe use of medicines
- be an invaluable point of reference for medical and pharmacy students.

There are also editions of the book aimed at dentists and nurse prescribers.

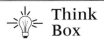 **Think Box**

Now most hospital docs don't wear nice white coats and walk around like they've escaped from a charity shop, where do they put the BNF?

NATIONAL CLINICAL ASSESSMENT AUTHORITY

- www.ncaa.nhs.uk

NCAA
9th Floor
Market Towers
1 Nine Elms Lane
London SW8 5NQ
Tel: 020 7273 0850
Fax: 020 7273 0851

> ☺ Not a very salubrious part of town but it is close to a Rolls-Royce dealership, not too far from the Oval cricket ground and house prices are on the way up.

This happy band are one of those 'special health authorities' in pursuit of the NHS holy grail:

quality

The NCAA have only been going since April 2003 so they are still finding which way up they are.

> **Think Box**
>
> I've never understood the NHS's approach to quality. It rewards quality and makes a big thing of it. In the real world, outside the NHS, quality is the foundation stone of business life. Poor quality – no business. It's as simple as that. Poor quality is punished. Good quality is a given.

They are aiming to sort out the performance of individual doctors, when PCOs, Trusts and community trusts have a problem.
   They will:

- provide advice
- carry out assessments.

It's too early to say how they will really work and how they will go about their business. They will publish detailed guidance in the autumn of 2003. So hold your breath and watch this space.

Think Box

This is interesting. They say they intend to have a *big involvement with the public*. Whether that means the usual suspects – patient groups and the like – or it means 'real' members of the real public remains to be seen. Remember, the majority of the real public have nothing to do with the NHS. Despite the huge numbers the NHS caters for, it is still a minority audience. Watch this space.

They say they are not destined to become a regulator. Rather, they will be supportive and provide advice on: 'how, and under what circumstances, health authorities and hospital and community trusts will be able to refer a dodgy doctor to the NCAA for assessment'.

They intend to: 'help the employer or health authority by carrying out an objective assessment. Following such an assessment, it will advise the trust or health authority on what to do next.'

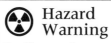 **Hazard Warning**

It all sounds very 'touchy-feely' to me!

Find out more about the background by taking a week off and reading this lot:

- *Supporting Doctors, Protecting Patients*
- *Assuring the Quality of Medical Practice: Implementing Supporting Doctors, Protecting Patients.*

Depending on your bandwidth, clog up your computer by downloading the reports from:

- www.doh.gov.uk/assuringquality

By the way, the NCAA only covers England and docs working in the prison service, but not Welsh docs and not dentists.

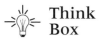 **Think Box**

By the way, the NCAA has no teeth. It can only recommend, and won't interfere with any of the rights and responsibilities of trusts, health authorities and doctors. So, what's the point? Dunno. Over to you!

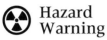 Hazard
Warning

It is likely that assessors will be drawn initially from the existing pool of individuals with the necessary skills. Does that mean mates assessing mates, old colleagues, friends and people they were at medical school with?

Whilst you think about it, bear in mind:

- the NCAA doesn't replace any of the existing complaints arrangements
- the emergence of the NCAA does not change the arrangements for referrals to the General Medical Council
- it interferes with the work of CHI and of its successor, CHAI.

OK, over to you . . .

Confused? Ring up the chairman, Mrs Jane Wesson, and ask her. Her number is: 020 7273 0850.

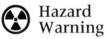 Hazard
Warning

In truth this is a tricky job in a minefield of vested and established interests. They will have to tiptoe through very carefully . . .

NHS Direct

All you need to know is the telephone number:

0845 4647

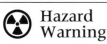 **Hazard Warning**

Yes, it's a short number. All calls are answered with a very irritating recorded voice about the Data Protection Act – there's friendly for you!

Welcome to the brave new world of healthcare: 24/7 on-the-phone help at the touch of a button.

Well, not quite. NHS Direct has a 98% approval rating amongst the patients who have used it. However, the GPs seem universally to hate it. They seem to think it doesn't reduce their workload. Rather, it increases it.

The scenario goes something like this: the worried well ring NHS Direct; the nurse taking the call is not too sure what is wrong and does the only safe thing they can – advises the caller to go and see a doctor.

On the other hand a bit of reassurance and advice to a worried mum is no bad thing. NHS Direct is the future and is yet to make its mark – but it will.

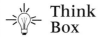 **Think Box**

The gods of Whitehall describe NHS Direct as a new gateway to healthcare. Do we need a new gateway? Answers on a postcard . . .

Call centres are the future for all kinds of service industry and there is no reason why the NHS should be any different.

NHS Direct will do this:

- tell you what to do if you're feeling ill
- give you advice about health concerns for you and your family
- tell you about local health services
- advise on self-help and support organisations.

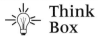 **Think Box**

An unnecessary addition to the NHS range of services or a first step into an uncertain future?

What do you think?

Have you tried it? What is your experience? Give 'em a test. Ring 'em up and ask them for the address and phone number of the late night pharmacy in your area. They should know!

NHS DIRECT ONLINE

Have a look at:

* www.nhsdirect.nhs.uk/

That's all there is to say, really. Have a look. Loadsa information. In the nooks and crannies of the NHS there are a number of interesting initiatives starting to show their green shoots.

☺ You can't write about a web service. Can you?

The NHS Information Authority, the big anoraks who are sorting out NHS IT, seem a bit nervous about the thousand flowers and are proposing a single gateway for all these websites. Makes sense, but it'll need to be a big portal and have a very clear front page.

NHS Direct Online claims to provide a gateway to good information and only links to high quality Internet information sources.

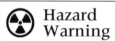

Hazard Warning

In November 1999, the *British Medical Journal* estimated there were something in the region of 100,000 health-related sites on the Internet.
How many of them are any good is anyone's guess.

The website has a helpline. So, if in doubt you can speak to a nurse on 0845 4647.
Recognise the number? Yup, it's NHS Direct. Interesting, eh?

CAREDIRECT

Another 'direct' . . . not very original, is it?

• www.doh.gov.uk/caredirect/text/home.htm

☺ This is a service dedicated to the needs of the over 60s. So, if you don't need it now, you will one day!

Ring Freephone CAREdirect on 0800 444 000 to find out about:

• pensions, benefits and other money matters
• care and support
• home issues
• health issues
• organisations that can help with all sorts – but probably not the address of the late night off-licence!

You will never believe the number of organisations it's taken to set this up! Try this list for size:

• Age Concern
• Association of Directors of Social Services
• Carers National Association
• Community District Nursing Association
• Help the Aged
• Housing Corporation
• Local Government Association
• National Centre for Independent Living
• National Housing Federation
• Royal College of Nursing
• Royal National Institute for the Blind
• UK Home Care Association.

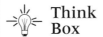

Think Box

Can anything involving this many organisations work?

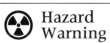

Hazard Warning

A note of caution: this is a pilot programme and is only live in part of the South-west of England. The plan is to cover the whole of England in the next four years or so.

THE NHS IN ENGLAND: THE BASICS

The NHS has just undergone yet another major shake-up in the way it is managed. That's the twelfth one I can remember! So what's new?

A cynic would say: nothing!

In the early years of the Thatcher Government there was a Richard Branson figure. He was called Griffiths and had a background in successful business. They hauled him in to have a look at why the NHS wasn't working, costing a fortune and going nowhere.

His advice was the NHS was being run by doctors and nurses who were very good at being doctors and nurses, but not much good at managing things. So Griffiths' advice was: the NHS needs an injection of competent management.

That was then, this is now!

This latest shake-up seems to be saying the NHS would be better run by doctors and nurses, as they know, better than managers, what patients need.

Ho, hum . . .

HERE'S HOW IT'S GOING TO WORK

Each year the money will be sent from the Treasury to the Department of Health and onto the Primary Care Organisations, who will be responsible for at least 70% of the local health economies (growing to nearly 100%). They will commission services from GPs (in effect themselves), Trust hospitals, the private sector or just about anyplace the quality is up to the job and the price is right.

They will work within a strategic framework, overseen by Strategic Health Authorities (StHAs).

WHAT'S NEXT?

- Foundation Hospitals with very significant freedom to manage their affairs, borrow money and engage staff on local pay and conditions.
- More devolution of power to Primary Care Organisations.
- More use of the private sector as service providers.
- A coming together of health and social service provision.

> ☺ All you need to know is that the changes are supposed to bring the management of the NHS closer to the patient. Sounds good!

THE STRUCTURE FOR BEGINNERS

Don't be shy, we all have to start somewhere, so why not here?

The Department of Health is in charge of the management and policy direction of the NHS in England. There has been a bit of organisation-shuffling, bringing together the Department of Health and the NHS Executive.

The old NHS Executive all got the sack and the DoH sits at the centre, lobbing out the cash and managing and setting standards and targets.

> ✓ For a nice picture of the structure of the NHS, try www.doh.gov.uk/codes/map.htm.

The next layer of management is the Strategic Health Authority.

Strategic Health Authorities were born of the thinking in a publication called *Shifting the Balance of Power*, an exciting little number that can be found at

- www.doh.gov.uk/shiftingthebalance/index.htm

> ☺ You need to know that from April 2003 the Department of Health's eight NHS regional offices were trashed and four new Regional Directors of Health and Social Care will be responsible for the development of the NHS. They will provide the link between the NHS organisations and the Government. Big, tough, influential jobs for some lucky boys and girls!

To save you the trouble, the idea is to give the power in the NHS to the frontline staff who understand patients' needs the best.

Local Primary Care Trusts (PCTs), increasingly known as Primary Care Organisations (PCOs), are the engine room of the NHS, assessing needs, planning and commissioning health services, and improving the health of residents in their localities.

Next comes NHS Trusts, who will provide secondary care and specialist services in hospitals – nothing much new there.

PLANNING HEALTH SERVICES IN ENGLAND

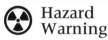 OK, listen up, this is really important. If you want to engage with the NHS in England you have to know this. Engage? Well, it's a sort of a euphemism for 'sell the NHS some of your stuff, flog 'em consultancy, goods, services or just the power of your mighty brain'. Knowing about all this will put you ahead of the game.

Unlike most of your other customers, the NHS is very transparent about what it intends to do and publishes its plans way up-front.

> ☺ Find out about all this and you have a ready-made marketing programme, all ready to impress your boss!

The Department of Health has developed a new planning framework, delivering a new three-year planning cycle for health and social care.

> ☢ **Hazard Warning**
>
> A three-year cycle? Doesn't the NHS plan year-on-year? No! Not any more. The Treasury changed the rules. The NHS knows three years in advance what its funding is going to be. In turn, that means they can plan service delivery and changes over a longer timescale. This makes for smoother transition and longer lead times into new projects. It's the kind of grown-up planning that the private sector has been doing for years.

This is good news and bad. The good news is: you can easily find out what your customers are up to and make a decision about how you want to engage with them.

It also means that if you miss the boat in year one, you'll be standing on the quayside for a good few years, waiting to get on board. The upshot is: you must get your field staff and road warriors to find out exactly what's in these plans – they are called:

Local Delivery Plans (LDPs)

Make a note: 'LDPs – mega important' and underline it twice!

Detailed guidance explaining this new planning framework and the processes that underpin it was issued to Strategic Health Authority (StHA) directors of planning on 8 November 2002. Find it on the DoH website:

www.doh.gov.uk

☺ Sometimes the abbreviation 'PCT' is changed to 'Primary Care Organisation' or 'PCO'.

It is all about roles and responsibilities for PCTs and builds on the Planning & Priorities Framework (PPF) guidance which was issued on 2 October 2002. Find it on the same website: www.doh.gov.uk.

The idea is for PCOs/PCTs to take the best experience of whole systems planning and cross-sector partnerships based on sound analysis of local needs, to build up the new Local Delivery Plans (LDPs) and any additional PCT-owned local plans.

LDPs will focus on the health and social care priorities set out in the PPF and will be the only formal plan requirement. They will be collated by StHAs and aggregated up into a report for the Health Authority area.

Primary Care Trusts (PCTs) have the key role in representing the NHS in local strategic planning arrangements around health improvement and inequalities and the development of partnerships with key local agencies.

This is significant and the planners have come up with a new word:

> This [role] will be *articulated* through local PCT strategic plans, as well as participation in Local Strategic Partnerships, other linked partnership arrangements and health chapters in Community Strategies.

Articulated! Got it? In other words, expressed or spoken. Other than the targets outlined in the PPF, arrangements for delivery will be a matter for local determination.

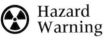 Hazard
Warning
There will, therefore, no longer be a formal requirement for PCTs to produce Health Improvement & Modernisation Plans (HImPs).

Pity really, because there is a very good book on how to write a HImP. It is published by the same publisher as this book and modesty prevents me from revealing the name of the author . . . Anyway, moving quickly on, LDPs are a sort of HImP, with knobs on.

The spirit of the HImP lives on; PCTs have the freedom to determine whether they want to develop any further plans covering locally agreed planning priorities that are non-PPF issues.

In case all this whizzo planning starts to take on the look of incomprehensible data, PCTs may present their local strategic planning in a more integrated form, which is 'more readily understandable for local partners and agencies, thereby aiding local joined-up delivery'. So sayeth the guidance on the topic.

In their appearance and structure the LDPs will look very much like the old HImP. They will cover:

- key health improvement issues drawn from national priority areas for locality (some may already feature in the LDP)
- local priorities for PCT action agreed through partnership arrangements.

> ☺ That's the key bit and this is the document you need to get hold of to find out what's happening on the ground. The age of the national marketing plan is dead. Enter the age of the very localised plan. Marketing managers need to be sure they have a nice new shelf in their office, all ready for the several hundred local plans that the local guys and girls will be sending you.

> ☺ In other words, this is where the bright and the best will spot new services emerging and be able to decide if they have any products and services that might help in their development and planning.

PCTs are told to make sure the HImP/LDP is able to align the health chapters in the Community Strategy *(a planning document that local authorities have to write, all very 'joined-up-government')* as part of the local picture and be appropriate for, and understandable to, an Overview & Scrutiny Committee and public involvement. So that means an easy to read and understand plan, ready to be turned into a sales development plan for you!

PCTs deal with a lot of other organisations and have to work flexibly with them and other partnerships, in particular local government, which operates on a different geography and time cycle to some PCTs.

This means the 'C' word: collaboration, to optimise local health organisations' and partners' capacity to deliver action on health improvement, particularly the national health inequalities targets, and contribute to neighbourhood renewal.

> ☀ **Think Box**
>
> All these arrangements need to be decided locally. It's big stuff, important, and you can see why a national plan, for a company wanting to engage with PCTs, is out of the window. Anyone who asks you to write a national marketing plan is living in the gas-lamp age. You'll have to rethink.

Community Strategies provide a means of rationalising partnerships as well as mechanisms and processes for engaging with local communities and the voluntary sector. There are clear, common aims, objectives and activity between the NHS and local government, many of which contribute to delivering NHS priorities.

A number of PCT and local authorities have already got their heads around this and the DoH are very keen that this development is supported across the whole country. PCTs are playing an important role in commanding both the lion's share of the local health economy and alignment with other organisations. But be warned: this varies from PCT to PCT, localities are in different stages of partnership development with their local government partners.

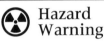 Hazard
Warning

For the umpteenth time *(sorry, no apology)*, you have to know what is going on locally. Variations can be found even a few miles down the road.

The actual process used for engagement with partners varies and is dependent on the variety of stakeholders in the health system, but the process of achieving partner involvement must be transparent. So keep in touch on the ground and you can easily find out what's going on.

In the words of the guidance oracle:

> Through this process, health partnerships are developing comprehensive local programmes with action across partnerships to improve health, tackle inequalities, and modernise the NHS. Involvement in the planning, prioritisation and delivery of strategic planning ensures that the stakeholders share ownership of NHS planning objectives.

So now you know and no excuses!

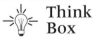 Think
Box

Just in case you think I've made too much of the importance of scrapping national and getting local, think for a moment: the PCOs control over 70% (and rising) of the cash in the local health economy, they determine referrals and patient flows, they supplement GP services wherever GPs opt out of service provision under the new contract, and they are the ringmaster in determining the shape of local services. Got the picture?

So make a note: get hold of the Local Delivery Plans – or die . . .

THE NHS IN NORTHERN IRELAND

Here's the web address you need:

• www.dhsspsni.gov.uk/index.html

and also . . . at www.n-i.nhs.uk/.

Just like the rest of the NHS in the British Isles, Northern Ireland has its fair share of change fever.

Add to that the general problems there about banging the heads of politicians together to make the place safe to live in and you can see the problem.

Many of the proposed reforms and changes have had to be shelved.

However, here's how it works at the moment. The Department of Health, Social Services and Public Safety, the boss organisation, is responsible for:

• health and personal social services, policy and legislation for hospitals, family practitioner services, community health and personal social services

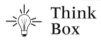 **Think Box**

They have the usual bit of motherhood-and-apple-pie, with a 'mission to improve the health and social well-being of the people of Northern Ireland'. What else would they do?

• public health, legislation to promote and protect the health and well-being of the population of Northern Ireland
• public safety, policy and legislation for the Fire Authority, food safety and emergency planning

. . . so good luck with all that!

✓ Organisationally they have a three-tier structure, a five-year, rolling Corporate Strategic Plan and 12 corporate strategic objectives, three French hens, two turtle doves and a partridge in a pear tree! It's all on the website. Plus the usual stuff; targets and all that.

Around the time the NHS in England was doing its thing, publishing its modernisation agenda, modernisation fever swept across the Irish Sea and evolved into a document published in March 1999, *Fit for the Future: A New Approach*, that set out the Government's proposals for the future of the health and personal social services in Northern Ireland.

In short, they set up the Department of Health, Social Services and Public Safety. Its job is:

- Health and Personal Social Services, which includes policy and legislation for hospitals, family practitioner services, community health and personal social services *(What else would it do?)*
- Public Health, which covers responsibility for policy and legislation to promote and protect the health and well-being of the population of Northern Ireland
- Public Safety, which will encompass responsibility for the policy and legislation for the Fire Authority, food safety and emergency planning. *(Mmmm, there's a lot I could say but I doubt the editor will let me! – Correct. Ed.)*

 Think Box

NHS anoraks will spot that there is an interesting difference in NI. Both health and social care is looked after by one Government department. Now that does make sense!

NHS anoraks will spot that there is an interesting difference in NI. Both health and social care is looked after by one government department. Now that does make sense!

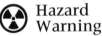 **Hazard Warning**

However, there is a catch. The 'health' bit of the Department doesn't raise taxes and relies on the conventional Exchequer grant system, unlike the social services bit, which gets its money from local government. Hence there is a mismatch in funding and they still have 'bed-blocking' and other problems, just like the rest of us.

The Department is run by a Permanent Secretary and the rest looks like this:

- the Planning and Resources Group, which does finance, staff, IT and all the usual stuff, plus: public health and safety policies, ambulance services, fire services and emergency planning; preparation and publication of the strategic plan for the health service – *so it is very busy!*

- HPSS Management Group for operational policy, performance management of Health and Personal Social Services and, as they put it, 'for ensuring its efficient and effective delivery'
- five professional groups, each one with a Chief Professional Officer: Medical and Allied Services, Social Services Inspectorate, Nursing and Midwifery Advisory Group, Pharmaceutical Advice and Services and Dental Services. Buried in here somewhere is also advice to the prison service.

> ☺ The Department currently employs about 850 staff and there are over 41,000 staff in the health and social services sector.

There is also an Occupational Health Service (OHS), the Employment Medical Advisory Service (part of the Health and Safety Executive for Northern Ireland) and Health Estates.

NEW LOCAL HEALTH AND SOCIAL CARE GROUPS

Sounds familiar? Well it is. It is very like the new English model. Fifteen new Local Health and Social Care Groups will be based around GP practices, 'and represent . . . natural communities, enabling local GPs and other primary care professionals to work in partnership with Boards, Trusts and local people to improve health and social services for the whole community'. Heard that before? Of course you have.

They will have six Groups in the Eastern Board area, four in the Northern Board, three in the Southern Board and two in the Western Board. There are huge ranges in the populations they cover. Even taking into account some awkward geography, it is still a big variation – between 60,000 to 200,000.

Here is the breakdown:

- Antrim/Ballymena: pop. 110,000
- Ards: pop. 71,000
- Armagh & Dungannon: pop. 103,000
- Causeway (Coleraine, Ballymoney and Moyle): pop. 97,000
- Craigavon & Banbridge: pop. 121,000
- Down: pop. 63,000.
- East Antrim (Larne, Carrickfergus and Newtownabbey): pop. 151,000

- Lisburn: pop. approx. 112,000
- Mid-Ulster (Magherafelt and Cookstown): pop. 70,000
- Newry & Mourne: pop. 87,000
- North & West Belfast: pop. approx. 155,000
- North Down: pop. 76,000
- Northern Group (Derry, Limavady and Strabane): pop. 164,000
- South & East Belfast: pop. 200,000
- Southern Group (Omagh and Fermanagh): pop. 118,000.

✓ Make a note: The Hayes Report.

Why make a note? Because it is controversial and proposes radical change. Written by a very Big Cheese, the chairman of the Acute Hospitals Review Group and former ombudsman Dr Maurice Hayes, and published in June 2001, it proposes:

- a new acute hospital to be built in County Fermanagh to serve the Southwest region
- the removal of accident and emergency services from five existing smaller acute hospitals

> ☺ The aim is to 'provide a seamless service where patients can move easily from primary care, easily through all the services they need'.

- rationalisation of hospital administration by replacing the four health boards with one 'strategic commissioning authority'
- merging the 18 hospitals trusts into three 'integrated health systems'.

The report recommends that three more hospitals should be added to the original six.

The original six are:

- the Royal Victoria and City Hospitals in Belfast
- the Ulster Hospital outside Belfast

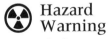 **Hazard Warning**
Try and close anything and you can expect a punch-up!

- Antrim Area Hospital in County Antrim
- Altnagelvin in County Londonderry
- Craigavon in County Armagh.

The report recommends the Causeway Hospital in Coleraine, County Londonderry, Daisy Hill Hospital in Newry, County Down, and a new Southwest hospital in Enniskillen should become acute centres.

As with all these brilliant reviews, there are winners and losers. The hospitals which would lose accident and emergency services would be the:

- County Antrim
- Lagan Valley, Lisburn
- Mater, Belfast
- Omagh, County Tyrone.

Oh, and for good measure, Whiteabbey Hospital in Newtownabbey, County Antrim, and the Downe and Downpatrick Hospitals would lose their maternity services.

Apparently the South Tyrone hospital in Dungannon, presently closed, would stay shut. The remaining hospitals will be merged into three super-trusts:

- Greater Belfast, including: the Royal, Belfast City, Musgrave Park, Mater, Ulster, Whiteabbey, Lagan Valley and Downe hospitals
- Northern, including: Altnagelvin, Antrim, Coleraine, Antrim and Coleraine
- Southern, including: Craigavon, Daisy Hill and the new Southwest hospital.

The report recommends doubling the number of hospital consultants and increasing the number of GPs by 25%. It does not suggest which page from the Harry Potter book of magic spells will be used to make this miracle happen. For good measure it has also annoyed the medical profession by suggesting a rotation system for doctors between the acute and local hospitals.

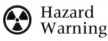 **Hazard Warning**

Expect the Mother of All Battles. I can't think of a hospital closure programme anywhere in the world that doesn't bring out the placard wavers and get the middle-classes waging war with their word processors!

Oh, and for the politicians who are working towards a united Ireland the Big Cheese suggests more cross-border co-operation on health.

The timescale for all this is 15 years. Yes, 15 years! Far too long to be measured and far too long to hold anyone to account. So: dreams, daft, waste of time, or a solid look into the future with realistic timescales?

Your call.

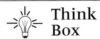 **Think Box**

Why is it so difficult to get the public to agree with NHS closures? They generally make eminent sense and end up providing better services. Is the NHS just poor at communication, or is there more to it than that?

THE NHS IN SCOTLAND

There only has to be a segment about healthcare in Scotland in this book because of devolution. Somehow we are to be persuaded that healthcare in Scotland is so different to the rest of the UK that it has to be run separately and funded separately, to employ people separately and be planned for separately.

> **Think Box**
>
> In health services terms, the whole of Scotland is only the size of an English region.

On the other hand, being able to get up close and personal with a region's healthcare may be no bad thing. As a result of the devolution programme, there is now a Scottish Parliament. There is also *loadsa* duplication between England and Scotland, in its institutions and planning.

The central management is by the Scottish Executive Health Department and Scotland is divided into 15 Area Health Boards and there are 28 self-governing NHS Trusts.

Nice and simple – yes. But, in the words of a great song: 'Then they go and spoil it all by doing something stupid like . . .' having Special Health Boards! For:

- health improvement and health promotion
- health protection
- needs assessment
- performance management of Trusts' implementation of Health Improvement Programmes
- resource allocation
- resource utilisation
- service development

. . . far too compartmentalised, if you ask me. *(No one is – Ed.)*

Healthcare is provided by Trust hospitals in the same way as in England. They can employ people on local terms and conditions, must work within budgets, plan healthcare in their areas, assess needs, be responsive, wear their underpants over their trousers and leap tall buildings in a single stride. All the usual stuff.

Trusts are run by:

- a non-executive Chairman appointed by the Secretary of State
- five executives, one of which is the Trust's Chief Executive
- five non-executive trustees.

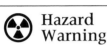 **Hazard Warning**

The non-executive trustees (it says in the paperwork), 'will be appointed to work as integral members of the management team'. That's potty; you can't be non-executive and be part of the management team. The whole idea is that the executive do the bidding of the non-executive. Looks like whoever wrote it had overdosed on motherhood-and-apple-pie!

. . . Just like England really!

There is another 'funny', too. Trusts have control of their estates but the Health Boards retain the responsibility for monitoring how it's used. Management gurus call this the 'holding on and letting go' dilemma that usually screws up good ideas.

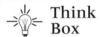 **Think Box**

By the way, there is something unique about the Scottish NHS: their Ambulance Service is the only nationwide (Scottish nation, that is) NHS Trust. They have annual service contracts with all 15 Health Boards and all 46 Hospital Trusts. This is obviously a dog's breakfast and the service has become a Special Health Board to deal with the bureaucracy.

The Health Boards look after that great management euphemism, 'strategic direction'. All based around something called Health Improvement Programmes, very important documents that are really the planning framework for the running and development of services.

✓ Anyone wanting to sell to the NHS in Scotland should treat these documents like a combination of the Bible, a marketing plan and the Holy Grail.

They are written to reflect local health needs and are reviewed annually.

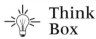 **Think Box**

There are about 132,000 staff in the Scottish NHS, 63,000 nurses, mid-wives and health visitors and over 8500 doctors. So they say. I've not counted them and I'm not sure they have either. Ask yourself the question. Sixty-three thousand nurses. Why not 63,020, or 62,999? Sixty-three thousand sounds too much like a nice round figure to be true!

There are also more than 7000 GPs. I couldn't tell you how many more there are but there are more than 7000! Plus all the usual dentists, opticians and community pharmacists, who are independent contractors.

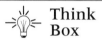 **Think Box**

Like most places, the Scottish health services struggle with a customer need based on a seamless interface between health and social services and a management and funding structure based on the two services being separate. The tartan solution is to publish a discussion paper on the relationship between these services. Watch this space, but not whilst holding your breath!

Just to make our lives difficult, there are two different types of Trust:

- Primary Care Trusts (PCTs), responsible for primary, community and mental health services within the geographical boundary of individual Health Boards (*coterminous boundaries – good idea!*)
- Acute Hospital Trusts (AHTs), responsible for a defined set of acute hospital services within the geographical boundary of individual Health Boards (*otherwise known as hospitals*).

Primary Care Trusts may also manage some hospital services, look after local services for people with learning disabilities, for people with mental health needs and the frail elderly.

☺ It is the Primary Care Trusts that have the principal role in delivering and planning healthcare needs – just like in England!

PCTs do all the usual stuff: support general practice; formulate primary care policy; direct the future development of services; work in partnership with

Health Boards, Acute Hospital Trusts and others to develop Health Improvement Programmes; implement local health strategies through Local Health
Care Co-operatives; deliver Trust Implementation Plans; engage primary and
secondary care clinicians in forming agreements on the design and delivery
of clinical services, reinforced through the allocation of Joint Investment
Funds; stimulate improvements in quality and standards of clinical care . . .
Give up?

Well, you get the picture. The PCTs run the show.

Funding of primary care under PCTs has the same intention as in England.
A move away from the individual practice model towards a collective
arrangement managed through the Local Health Care Co-operatives.

Co-operatives can hold a budget for primary and community health
services if they wish. This is new and is the subject of a Government
review to see how it works.

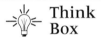 **Think
Box**

They do have a neat idea: Local Health Care Co-operatives. Made up of
voluntary organisations of GPs, they take a wider view on such imperatives as: working with public health professionals to develop plans which
reflect the clinical priorities for an area; population-wide approaches to
health improvement and disease prevention which require lifestyle and
behavioural change *(Sounds like the Health Police! No deep-fried Mars Bars for
you, wee laddie!)*; and improving the quality and standards of clinical care
through professional development, education, training, research and
audit.

One very good tartan idea is Joint Investment Funds. They take all the
money that is spent on a disease area and view it as a global budget to
see if it could be better utilised. Excellent! So, for example, the management of CHD patients, often in both the primary and secondary sector, is
seen as one patient experience and the money 'invested' in the model of
care most likely to benefit the patient. Very good! Diseases don't
recognise the difference between primary and secondary care, so why
should money?

☺ As if by magic, the number of Acute Hospital Trusts in Scotland has
been reduced, they say for 'greater efficiency to be secured through
elimination of duplication and wasteful competition'. Mmmm, nice one.

The aim in most Health Board Areas of having one Acute Hospital Trust has been achieved, except in Glasgow.

The patient voice is listened to via Local Health Councils. They get involved in:

- changes in the pattern of service which are to be achieved
- resources which the Board intends to make available
- the expected level of service to be delivered.

However they do it, it looks like it works!

There are 15 Health Board Areas:

- Argyll and Clyde Health Board Area
- Ayrshire and Arran Health Board Area
- Borders Health Board Area
- Dumfries and Galloway Health Board Area
- Fife Health Board Area
- Forth Valley Health Board Area
- Grampian Health Board Area
- Greater Glasgow Health Board Area
- Highland Health Board Area
- Lanarkshire Health Board Area
- Lothian Health Board Area
- Orkney Health Board Area *(Great place for a holiday. I know – I've been there!)*
- Shetland Health Board Area
- Tayside Health Board Area
- Western Isles Health Board Area.

THE NHS IN WALES

OK, I've got to be honest. I find it hard to get excited about the fact the NHS in Wales is 'different'. It looks to me like they have the same stuff as in England but it all comes with a dragon on the cover.

So, that will have annoyed the *$&& out of all the Welsh readers, now let's have a closer look at NHS Wales . . .

- It provides comprehensive care.
- Everyone has the right to use it.
- Care is provided on the basis of people's clinical need – not on their ability to pay.

Not too much different there, then? Just laver bread and apple pie.

The National Assembly for Wales is responsible for policy direction and for allocating funds to the NHS, but it can't raise taxes.

> ☺ The NHS is Wales' largest employer, with 60,000 staff, representing more than 7% of the Welsh workforce.

The future of the NHS in Wales is under review. Like everywhere else, they have a dose of modernisation fever. They have a document called *Structural Change in the NHS*. Not very sexy, but businesslike.

Full details can be found at:

- www.wales.gov.uk/healthplanonline/newsletter/struc_consul_report_e.htm

It includes phrases such as: 'challenges, new approaches, dynamic partnerships and strong leadership'. Oh, and 'clear accountabilities at all levels'. Yawn . . .

The upshot of this is that there will be Local Health Boards (LHBs) in every area, serving their own localities. *(If it sounds like PCT in England, it is because they are the same thing.)*

LHBs will provide a local focus for the development and improvement of health services. They will 'decide what services are needed for local people and make sure that these are provided'.

They will do that by:

- developing Health Improvement Programmes (HImPs)
- developing the principles of clinical governance to improve the quality of primary healthcare
- informing and developing the commissioning of hospital and community health services.

Local Health Boards will be made up of:

- local doctors
- nurses
- other health professionals
- representatives from the local Council (including elected members)
- voluntary organisations
- the public.

And something (at last) a bit different: a carer will sit on every Board.

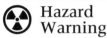 **Hazard Warning**

As in Northern Ireland and Scotland, in the new Welsh system, local government and Local Health Boards will work together more closely, so that there is better co-ordination of services, especially health and social services. Why they don't merge the services is still a mystery.

NHS Trusts will continue to run hospitals and community services.

Services which are too specialised to be dealt with locally will continue to be organised on an all-Wales basis for delivery in all parts of Wales.

You can keep up to date with all the changes at:

- www.wales.gov.uk/healthplanonline/newsletter/index.htm

There is a helpful directory at:

- www.wales.nhs.uk/org.cfm

To save you browsing, you might like to know that in Wales there are about 1900 family doctors, around 1000 dentists and 600 opticians. And there are 15 NHS Trusts, including one pan-Wales ambulance trust. These Trusts manage 135 hospitals with some 15,000 beds. So, now you are an expert!

☺ Unlike in England, where the Community Health Councils have been dumped, Welsh NHS Trusts and Health Authorities are required by law to consult their Community Health Council if they propose major changes in the pattern or provision of services. You will find a CHC in each of the 22 local government areas in Wales and they take up a wide range of health issues on behalf of the public. And they do a good job. I never understood why they got the chop in England.

The Health and Social Services Secretary in the National Assembly is the boss.

The Head of the NHS Directorate in the National Assembly is the civil servant responsible.

They have a Chief Medical Officer and the head of the Health Improvement and Protection Directorate in the National Assembly.

Having been very sceptical about the need for a difference between English and Welsh healthcare systems, I have to say the Welsh system does base its local health groups on the geography of the local authorities. Very sensible. The English system started out to do this and somehow lost the plot.

So, what about the Assembly? What does it do for health? Its powers are to:

- draw up strategic policies for health and health services and allocate resources
- configure the NHS in Wales in a way that is consistent with its broader objectives
- hold NHS organisations to account for their performance
- promote the provision of particular services in Wales.

Nothing very earth-shattering. For anoraks, the base-line document *The White Paper: Putting Patients First* can be downloaded at:

- www.wales.gov.uk/subihealth/content/keypubs/whitepaper/intro_e.htm

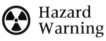 **Hazard Warning**
The preface to this fine example of truly historic writing is by the Prime Minister . . . So you'd better read it, 'cause when you meet him you can chat to him about it!

NHS SUPPLIES AUTHORITY (NOT THEIR PROPER TITLE, BUT I'LL GET TO THAT!)

This is where all the stuff comes from – from bandages to bread.

They live here *(and very grand it is, too!)*, but they have regional distribution centres all over the place:

NHS Supplies Authority
Premier House
60 Caversham Road
Reading RG1 7EB
Tel: 0118 980 8600
Fax: 0118 980 8650
www.supplies.nhs.uk

This is what they say they try to do:

> The Authority's principal role is to enable the NHS to obtain the maximum possible benefit from the money it spends on the goods and services it requires for the delivery of healthcare. The Authority aims to be the NHS's own supplies centre of expertise, knowledge and excellence.

Well, they are not without their critics and they have had a pretty controversial background.

This is what a committee of MPs said about them:

> Experience of establishing a central supplies organisation for the NHS in England has proved to be slow and to produce only modest savings. As a result healthcare providers have incurred unnecessary costs. The MPs doubt whether the move to a single purchasing organisation has been achieved with sufficient urgency.
>
> The NHS Supplies Authority came into being in 1991 to remove inefficiencies in the previous supply system managed by regional health authorities. Since then the authority has spent £8bn and made savings of £260m, which seem modest to the committee, particularly as the authority costs £70m a year to run.
>
> In view of these modest savings the committee is surprised that

the NHS Executive relaxed the savings targets for 1996–7. 'We expect the NHS Executive to take a hard look at the scope for further saving and to set tough targets for NHS supplies,' the committee concludes, adding that the operation should match best commercial practice.

The NHS Executive accepts the scope for further economies and forecast savings of £150m over three years.

In case you might like to try a little bedside reading, the above extract is from *NHS Supplies in England*, available from The Stationery Office, price £8. Or a system-clogging download from The Stationery Office website, if you have an account with them.

As a result of that and other criticisms from the Audit Commission and the forerunner to the NHS Confederation, the Federation of NHS Trusts, there was a shake-up. It got complicated.

Here's how the supplies guys (and girls) describe it on their website.

NHS PURCHASING AND SUPPLY AGENCY – THIS IS THEIR PROPER TITLE!

The NHS Purchasing and Supply Agency is an executive agency of the Department of Health, established on 1 April 2000.

Formed as a result of recommendations contained in the Cabinet Office Review of NHS Procurement (published in June 1999) the Agency, together with its sister organisation the NHS Logistics Authority, replace the Special Health Authority NHS Supplies.

Here is a bit of the history . . .

NHS Supplies was formed in 1991 as the purchasing and supply arm of the NHS in England. Their job was to achieve the best value for money for the NHS on the goods and services it purchased. The organisation operated through three business divisions – Customer Services, Purchasing and Wholesaling.

OK, back to the NHSPSA website. Now they describe what happened next:

- the establishment of the NHS Purchasing and Supply Agency to act as a strategic advisor to the NHS on supply issues. The

agency was formed from NHS Supplies' Purchasing Division
and some corporate functions
- a separate logistics operation for the NHS – the NHS Logistics
Authority – formed from NHS Supplies' Wholesaling Division
- the transfer of staff from NHS Supplies' Customer Services
Division – which provided dedicated supplies staff based
on-site at individual Trusts – to the employment of their
host Trust. This was completed by the end of October 1999.

OK, so what does this spanking new outfit do?

The role of the new agency is to act as a centre of expertise,
knowledge and excellence in purchasing and supply matters for
the health service. As an integral part of the Department of
Health, the NHS Purchasing and Supply Agency is in a key
position to advise on policy and the strategic direction of
procurement, and its impact on developing healthcare, across
the NHS.

Intended to function not just as an advisory and co-ordinating
body but also an active participant in the ongoing modernisation
of purchasing and supply in the health service, the agency
contracts on a national basis for products and services which
are strategically critical to the NHS. It also acts in cases where
aggregated purchasing power will yield greater economic savings
than those achieved by contracting on a local or regional basis.

The agency works with around 400 NHS Trusts and health
authorities and manages 3000 national purchasing contracts,
influencing around half of the £7 billion spent in the NHS on
purchasing goods and services in the health service.

The common law of business logic is: 'the more you buy, the cheaper it gets'.
It's not quite that simple in the NHS.

Think about it. The NHS buys millions of bits and pieces, from the most
complex medical equipment to bog rolls. That requires an extraordinary
diversity of expertise.

Then there is the logistics bit. This is
tough. They buy in bulk and break con-
signments down to fulfil the requirements
of their customers – the NHS Trusts. That
means handling and that means costs.

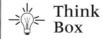

Think Box

So, there is a problem. Have
they got it sorted?

Few hospitals have got really efficient stores, efficient in the sense of being like out-the-back in Sainsbury's. Even fewer hospitals are designed for proper just-in-time delivery. And just-in-time is as much a product of building design as anything else.

The NHSPSA do come in for some stick over their on-costs. Many claim these are too high and put an artificial premium on the cost of supplies to the NHS. Others say it is complex business and they play a bad hand very well. Comparisons with the likes of Sainsbury's, Tesco and Marks and Sparks make the NHSPSA's on-costs look high.

The question is: is it a fair comparison?

There is no obligation on NHS Trusts and other establishments to buy from the NHSPSA. Indeed, it is quite the reverse. The NHSPSA competes for business. There are other, private sector suppliers who can provide for some of the requirements of NHS Trusts. There is an obligation on NHS Trusts to demonstrate that they are getting as many bangs for the taxpayers' bucks as possible. As a consequence, something known as 'cherry picking' has emerged.

In short, 'cherry picking' describes what happens when Trusts purchase selected items direct from suppliers, who can sell them at a lower price than the NHSPSA charges for the same item. How does it work? It cuts out the middle-men and the on-costs of the NHSPSA. This is profitable for the suppliers, as the items go from their factory, direct to the Trust, without the added on-cost of the NHSPSA.

This infuriates the NHSPSA, as it undermines their role. But hard-pressed Trusts, worried about delivering on budget, have little option. Some suppliers claim they can sell to Trusts cheaper than they sell to the NHSPSA and still make a profit. Funny old world, ain't it?

Got products to sell to the NHS? If you want to get the lion's share of the market, develop hard knuckles and be prepared to spend a lot of time knocking on the NHSPSA's doors and expect a pretty bureaucratic procurement regime. But, once you are *in*, you are *in*.

Alternatives – sell direct to Trusts. Higher marketing costs but a faster penetration into the market.

Really stuck? I'm told a word in the shell-like ear-hole of your local MP about Soviet-style bureaucracy and jobs in the constituency can speed things up!

Good luck!

NHS INFORMATION AUTHORITY

Information technology, information systems, computing and joined-up hospitals and doctors.

> ☺ They live in rather commodious offices in Birmingham, but the car park is always full. If you are visiting, try to get a visitor's bay reserved or get there at about 5.30am!

NHS Information Authority
Aqueous II
Aston Cross
Rocky Lane
Birmingham B6 5RQ
Tel: 0121 333 0333 – it is a very fast switchboard, with a real person!
Fax: 0121 333 0334

And there is a rather disappointing website at:

* www.nhsia.nhs.uk

I'm not sure why I'm disappointed, it's just – well, IT and all that; I expected something a bit more song-and-dance.

This is what they say they do:

> To do what's best done nationally

Yup, their words not mine. Funny phrase? Well, you need a bit of an inside track to understand it. The NHS is something of an electronic Tower of Babel. There are hundreds of computer systems that have been plugged in over the years. Many of them are basket-cases developed by men who live in sheds and wear bobble hats.

When the NHS woke up to the fact it couldn't modernise diddly squat without sorting its IT out, it embarked on a piece of management madness called a 'local strategy, for local implementation'.

> 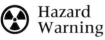 **Hazard Warning**
> The NHS abounds in IT products dreamt up by enthusiasts. Some of them are good but most of them are, er, shall we say esoteric . . .

You don't have to be a management guru to see the mess that got into. The NHSIA neatly tried to sidestep the problems, hence the cute little phrase. They are a bit more forthcoming. Here are their words:

> As a Special Health Authority, the NHS Information Authority has an established and overall remit to:
>
> 'Improve patient care and achieve best value for money (VFM) by working with NHS professionals, suppliers and academics and others to provide national products, services and standards, which support the sharing and most efficient and effective use of information.'
>
> This will be achieved by:
> - Building and maintaining an understanding of the problems we are helping to resolve using consultation techniques involving the public and patients
> - Enabling the NHS to use information to improve the quality of patient care
> - Aligning our delivery in accordance with healthcare priorities, such as National Service Frameworks
> - Creating a reputation for delivering products and services that satisfy stakeholder requirements.

There's more. There would have to be! A bland, generic mission statement like that wouldn't be worth hanging on the wall without a set of equally bland objectives!

> - Support the effective use of national electronic health records to improve patient care through the provision of the Integrated Care Record System (ICRS)
> - Provide information services and knowledge for decision-making for staff, patients and public
> - Establish and maintain Health Informatics as a recognised and respected national profession
> - Provide reliable and secure information infrastructure services
> - Provide specialist support services for national initiatives.

Still awake? Who writes this stuff?

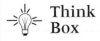 **Think Box**

You will note that in those two hundred or so words there is not one mention of a computer! My guess is they thought they might frighten the natives, used to a pencil and paper.

They seem to forget: most NHS staff have more computing power in their kids' bedrooms than they do on their office desks.

If this seems a bit of a mess, it is because it is. The Gods of Whitehall tried to sort it out and shuffled the job of oversight around the in-trays of Westminster. In the end they did the right thing – unusually! They bought themselves a Rottweiler.

Enter Richard Granger. Granger is the man who delivered the technical bits of the London Congestion Charge system – on time and in budget. Now the words 'on time and in budget' are a bit of a rarity in the public sector, but Granger did it.

He is tough, uncompromising, smart, hard-hitting, dangerous, blunt and never takes prisoners. In other words, he is very good news for the NHS, whose whole future depends on getting the best from IM&T.

As we go to press he's told the IT suppliers their fortune, frightened most NHS IT professionals half to death and made it pretty clear he will deliver the NHS IT agenda, on time and in budget. You know what? I believe him.

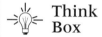

Think Box

I shouldn't worry too much about getting a parking space in Birmingham. In my view the NHSIA is set to become a fig-leaf for spending respectability and public accountability. The ones to watch are the Strategic Health Authorities charged with the performance management of IT implementation and the PCOs who will be given operational responsibility for primary care IT.

The days of flogging the docs a nice bit of software are over.

✓ Tip: get to meet Granger if you can!

NATIONAL INSTITUTE FOR CLINICAL EXCELLENCE (KNOWN TO ITS FRIENDS AS NICE)

They have a superb website at:

- www.nice.org.uk/

| NICE provides a service for the NHS in England and Wales. |

What is NICE all about? Rationing, putting a rationale behind the use of resources, finding out what is cost-effective and clinically effective, finding out what we should be spending our money on, a barrier to the entry of new medicines? Take your pick. Depends if you are a pharmaceutical manufacturer, doctor, manager or patient.

☺ You can register on their website, tell them what you are really interested in and as soon as there is something new, they'll send you an email to let you know. It's called 'push technology'. Neat, eh?

NICE is the NHS's most misunderstood child.

Set up in 1999, NICE is a pivotal part of the Government's modernisation agenda. NICE is a Special Health Authority and systematically appraises health interventions used in the NHS.

Manufacturers are given advanced notice that a product may be subject to appraisal – and companies are invited to submit evidence of clinical and cost-effectiveness.

NICE guidance is provided to help clinicians to use treatments that work best for patients. This includes guidelines for the management of certain diseases or conditions and guidance on the appropriate use of particular interventions.

 Think Box

It is frequently overlooked that the Department of Health in England and the National Assembly for Wales select the topics that NICE looks at.

Contrary to early expectations, NICE has said 'yes' to more interventions than it has said 'no' to. Indeed, it has added over £600m to the cost of the NHS's medicine cabinet. The Government has issued directions that have the effect of placing a statutory obligation on Health Authorities and Primary Care Trusts to provide appropriate funding for treatments recommended by NICE.

This is a headache for the Primary Care Trusts who have to juggle the budgets.

Here's how it's stacking up so far: £250 million was spent in 2002 on treatments recommended by NICE, including:

- £10 million on NICE-recommended drugs to treat cancers of the pancreas, lungs, brain and leukaemia, benefiting around 10,000 people
- £76 million on NICE's guidance on drugs and interventions for people with coronary heart disease, to the advantage of over 70,000 patients
- £30 million on funding NICE's appraisals of drugs to treat breast and ovarian cancer. This means around 9000 women have had faster and secure access to treatment.

NICE have an extensive work programme and the information on their website is very comprehensive.

If you don't know what's going on at NICE, it's your fault, or you've been living in a cave.

BRITISH MEDICAL ASSOCIATION

- www.bma.org.uk/

This is the doctors' trade union. They claim to have 123,000 plus members, including 4000 or so from overseas.

> ☺ They also have 12,000 medical students in membership. Nothing like getting 'em early!

The BMA does not register doctors; that is the job of the General Medical Council (GMC). Neither does it discipline doctors; that's the job of the employer or the GMC. Neither is it allowed to recommend doctors to members of the public.

If you'd like to visit them, you'll find them at some rather superbly appointed premises at:

British Medical Association
BMA House
Tavistock Square
London WC1H 9JP
Tel: 020 7387 4499 (head office)

> 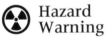 **Hazard**
> **Warning**
> Contrary to popular belief, membership of the BMA is not compulsory for doctors. About 20% of UK practising doctors do not belong.

Don't even think about driving there. Also, the security is better than the Pentagon. Once inside, nothing will prepare you for the lavish comfort and the atmosphere of relaxed cosiness.

> ☺ BMA, sometimes known as the British Machiavellian Army.

COUNCIL FOR THE REGULATION OF HEALTHCARE PROFESSIONALS

Another layer of bureaucracy. Their *raison d'être* is to co-ordinate and oversee the work of all the existing regulatory bodies. Quite why, I'm not too sure!

They say of themselves that they will: 'build and manage a new framework for self-regulation'.

There's a whole list of good intentions. They say they will:

- share good practice between the existing regulatory bodies
- work towards improved accountability and greater openness in the NHS. *(What does 'working towards' mean? Does it mean they'll ever get there?)*

Here's some more %^!!**. See what you think:

> The new Council will act as an overarching body which will oversee the individual regulators, but will not get involved in the direct regulation of healthcare professionals. Instead, it will ensure consistency in the work of the regulators. As a last resort, it will be able to require a regulator to change its rules in the public interest provided both Houses of Parliament agree.

Yeah, well . . .

How did all this come about? In the post-Shipman and Bristol NHS, anything is possible!

It will have nine members from the professions and ten representing public interests and the NHS.

The regulators they will be 'regulating' are:

- Council for Professions Supplementary to Medicine*
- General Chiropractic Council
- General Dental Council
- General Medical Council
- General Optical Council
- General Osteopathic Council
- Pharmaceutical Society of Northern Ireland
- Royal Pharmaceutical Society
- UK Central Council for Nursing, Midwifery and Health Visiting.*

* (and their successors, 'cause they are being shaken up, too)

GENERAL MEDICAL COUNCIL

- www.gmc-uk.org/

The big guns. Run by doctors for the benefit of doctors, a closed shop and a dinosaur? Or a thoughtful group of professionals keen to regulate their colleagues and focus on best practice?

   It is true the GMC went through a bad patch where they looked flat-footed and self-focused. They've been through a long consultation process and dusted themselves down and this is what they are saying about themselves:

> We have strong and effective legal powers designed to maintain the standards the public have a right to expect of doctors. We are not here to protect the medical profession – their interests are protected by others. Our job is to protect patients.

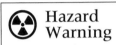 **Hazard Warning**
Mmmm. I have to confess, I come from the 'self-regulation-sucks' school of thinking.

>   The public trust doctors to set and monitor their own professional standards. In return doctors must give their patients high-quality medical care. Where any doctor fails to meet those standards, we act to protect patients from harm – if necessary, by striking the doctor off the register and removing their right to practise medicine.
>
>   We are a charity (registration number 1089278) whose purpose is the protection, promotion and maintenance of the health and safety of the community.

This is how they do all this good stuff.

   Their full Council meets only three times a year, in February, May and November. They claim most of their work is done in committees that meet throughout the year.

   They have 104 members: 54 doctors elected by the doctors on the register, 25 members of the public nominated by the Privy Council and 25 doctors appointed by educational bodies – the universities, medical royal colleges and faculties.

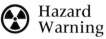
Hazard
Warning

I can hear you saying 'Privy Council?' Yup, I know. And look at the balance of numbers between the docs and their customers. Sorry, I just don't go for it.

If you agree or disagree with me, you can write and tell 'em at:

General Medical Council
178 Great Portland Street
London W1W 5JE

At the time of going to press the GMC is consulting on a new document, *New Arrangements for GMC Registration and Licensure: a consultation paper.*

You can get it/see it on their website. Unless you are of the chosen few, the great unwashed are not invited to comment. Nevertheless, it is worth a read. Send 'em a comment anyway – see what they do!

The GMC strapline is:

Protecting patients, guiding doctors.

. . . Nice one, puts the customer first and all that. Very Islington! I wonder whether it is the invention of a very good PR person or whether they really mean it?

There are about 208,000 medical practitioners registered with the GMC. Every year about 11,000 new entries appear on the register; 40% are newly qualified, bright-eyed and bushy-tailed UK graduates; 15% are docs who qualified elsewhere in the EEA and the rest – 45% – qualified outside Europe.

GENERAL SOCIAL CARE COUNCIL (GSCC)

* www.gscc.org.uk/

Same as the General Medical Council but for regulating the social care workforce through a code of conduct for employees, a code of practice for employers and by operating registers for sectors of the social care workforce.

Unlike the GMC, who have been around since God wore short trousers, this lot have only been going since 1 October 2001. It is the first ever regulatory body for the social care workforce in England. About time too. Let's wish 'em luck.

Its job is to:

* set codes of conduct and practice for social care workers and employers
* establish a register of 1.2 million social care workers
* regulate social work education and training.

It is accountable to the Secretary of State for Health.

You can call them on 020 7210 5375.

HEALTH PROTECTION AGENCY

This lot only got started on 1 April 2003.

To find out more you need to read a copy of a publication from January 2002 called *Getting Ahead of the Curve: A Strategy for Combating Infectious Diseases*.

The Chief Medical Officer got very excited and described the HPA as:

> one of the most exciting and innovative developments in the field of health protection for many years. In the face of new and continuing threats from infectious diseases and environmental hazards, the Agency will be able to provide more effective services for health protection and health emergency planning than the existing, more fragmented, arrangements.

That's all you need to know, really.

The report recommended combining the existing functions of the following national bodies:

- Centre for Applied Microbiology & Research
- National Radiological Protection Board
- Public Health Laboratory Service
- The National Focus for Chemical Incidents.

The report also recommended lumping together:

- Consultants in Communicable Disease Control
- Health Emergency Planning Advisors and Infection Control.

They will get out and about a bit, too. They will provide a *dedicated field service* and an *integrated approach* to protecting the public against infectious diseases and chemical and radiological hazards.

INSTITUTE OF HEALTHCARE MANAGEMENT

- www.ihm.org.uk/

If you are a manager in the NHS you should belong to this lot. They've been through some difficult days and a few incarnations but they are still around, expanded and speak for the very important group of NHS managers.

They have recently merged the Institute of Health Services Management and the Association of Managers in General Practice. It is the largest professional organisation for individual managers in all areas of healthcare.

This is what it says of itself:

> The Institute's purpose is:
> - to enhance and promote high standards of professional health-care management in order to improve health and healthcare for the benefit of the public.
>
> The IHM's major objectives are:
> - to create, sustain and represent a professional community of healthcare managers
> - to provide an independent voice for healthcare managers, and to protect and promote the status, interests and welfare of the members by ensuring that their contribution to good health and healthcare is recognised
> - to influence policy, operations and culture in UK healthcare
> - to provide strong local networks and support for members, especially in times of professional difficulty
> - to promote professional standard-setting
> - to promote good practice and professional development
> - to advance the study of and research in healthcare management
> - to provide/support the education of healthcare managers.

The Institute has recently developed a code of practice for managers and the talk is that it may become mandatory for all managers to subscribe to it. Otherwise – no job!

Members are drawn from primary care, secondary care, mental health and community care, including chief executives, middle managers and students from all sectors, whether public, private or voluntary.

They live at:

Institute of Healthcare Management
PO Box 33239
46 Grosvenor Gardens
London SW1W 0WN
Tel: 020 7881 9235
Fax: 020 7881 9236

KING'S FUND

• www.kingsfund.org.uk/

Once very pre-eminent in healthcare policy development and analysis.
More recently, perhaps, they appear to have lost their way.

The King's Fund is an independent charity with a very interesting history.
They aim to:

> . . . tackle health inequalities and social injustice, enabling health
> and social care staff and organisations to work in partnership,
> across traditional boundaries promoting cultural diversity in
> health encouraging patient and wider public involvement in
> health and healthcare.

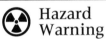 **Hazard**
Warning

They have some really nice offices. But they recently shut their bookshop,
which I take very personally! How a think tank/research organisation can
shut their bookshop baffles me. Perhaps it didn't sell enough books? It
does, however, have a very good library. Modesty prevents me from
telling you the name of one of the authors whose work you will find on
the shelves!

They are dependent on the income from an endowed block of investments.
The stock market has gone down the pan and so has a large slice of the
Fund's fund! There are all sorts of rumours about the future of the Fund and
the chief executive has, unexpectedly, announced her retirement. As we go
to press they are advertising for a successor.

Watch this space.

King's Fund
11–13 Cavendish Square
London W1G 0AN
Tel: 020 7307 2400
Fax: 020 7307 2801

LEADERSHIP PROGRAMME

• www.doh.gov.uk/about/nhsplan/who/modagency01.html#lp

☹ Another new initiative. The Leadership Programme's main purpose is to:

> . . . build the capacity of all managers in the NHS to fulfil their potential. The team commissions, develops and manages national programmes to develop leaders, working closely with the NHS, business schools and universities.

Mmmmmmmmmm . . .

NHS LEARNING NETWORK TEAM

- www.doh.gov.uk/about/nhsplan/who/modagency01.html#lnt

☹ Another initiative . . .

The 'Team' says it exists to 'streamline the sharing of information, intelligence, knowledge and know how'. For my money, simply stick it on a website. But this is the NHS. Nothing is simple.

There are four main elements to the Learning Network:

- good practice shared through beacons and NHS Learning Centres
- information exchange on good practice
- leadership
- management development.

In fairness, there *is* a website. Have a look at:

- www.doh.gov.uk/learningzone/index.htm

It provides:

- information about how NHS and non-NHS organisations have tried to improve service delivery for patients

> ☺ There are some external links, but beware: some links are not available to users who do not have NHSNet access.

- details of national programmes
- examples of best practice
- official guidance.

NHS ALLIANCE

• www.nhsalliance.targaweb.co.uk/index.html

Born of the NHS modernisation reforms, the Alliance emerged as a new organisation to represent the views of the new shape of primary care. The Alliance claims currently to represent three-quarters of English Primary Care Groups.

> ☺ It lobbies on behalf of its members and shares good practice.

Most of the organisation's members are individuals – GPs, nurses, Allied Health Professionals, managers and lay board members.

At present the head honcho is an enthusiastic GP who wears a bow-tie . . .

NHS Alliance
Retford Hospital
North Road
Retford
Notts DN22 7XF
Tel: 01777 869080
Fax: 01777 869081

NHS CONFEDERATION

- www.nhsconfed.net/
- www.nhsconfed.org/

 Think Box

The NHS Confederation is the only membership body for all NHS organisations. Because of this, some say they can't represent anyone. If they support an initiative in primary care that has a derogatory impact on secondary care their secondary care membership get upset. And vice versa. They say they 'connect the family' of the NHS. Nice line, good spin doctor, eh? What do you think? Can you represent everyone?

The NHS Confederation is a registered charity. Charity no: 283447. And their London office is at:

NHS Confederation
1 Warwick Row
London SW1E 5ER
Tel: 020 7959 7272
Fax: 020 7959 7273

They have a very smart way of letting you contact them. Got the name of the person you want to email? Here is the template:

- firstname.lastname@nhsconfed.co.uk

ORTHOPAEDIC SERVICES COLLABORATIVE

- www.doh.gov.uk/about/nhsplan/who/modagency01.html#osc

The Orthopaedic Services Collaborative is designed to allow all trauma and orthopaedic departments in England who want to improve their services to participate in modernisation programmes.

> ☺ Did you know about these good folk, beavering away? If you did, you either work for them, have a special interest in orthopaedics or are an irredeemable NHS anorak!

Involvement is on a voluntary basis.

ROYAL COLLEGES

Loads of them, going back for years. Stuck in the past, or established, reliable and sensible? No prizes for guessing what I think!
   Here's a selection to be going on with:

Royal College of Physicians of London
11 St Andrew's Place
Regent's Park
London NW1 4LE
Tel: 020 7935 1174
www.rcplondon.ac.uk/

Royal College of Radiologists
38 Portland Place
London W1N 4JQ
Tel: 020 7636 4432

Royal College of Physicians of Ireland
6 Kildare Street
Dublin 2
Ireland
Tel: +35 31 661 6677

Royal College of Psychiatrists
17 Belgrave Square
London SW1X 8PG
Tel: 020 7235 2351

Royal College of Obstetricians and Gynaecologists
27 Sussex Place
Regent's Park
London NW1 4QW
Tel: 020 7772 6200

Royal College of Physicians of Edinburgh
9 Queen Street
Edinburgh EH2 1JQ
Tel: 0131 225 7324

Faculty of Public Health Medicine
4 St Andrew's Place
Regent's Park
London NW1 4LB
Tel: 020 7935 0243

Royal College of Paediatrics and Child Health
50 Hallam Street
London W1N 6DE
Tel: 020 7307 5600
www.rcpch.ac.uk/

Royal College of General Practitioners
14 Princes Gate
London SW7 1PU
Tel: 020 7581 3232
www.rcgp.org.uk/

Royal College of Ophthalmologists
17 Cornwall Terrace
Regent's Park
London NW1 4QW
Tel: 020 7935 0702

Royal College of Anaesthetists
48/49 Russell Square
London WC1B 4JY
Tel: 020 7813 1900
www.rcoa.ac.uk/

Royal College of Pathologists
2 Carlton House Terrace
London SW1Y 5AF
Tel: 020 7451 6700

Royal College of Physicians and Surgeons of Glasgow
232–242 St Vincent Street
Glasgow G2 5RJ
Tel: 0141 221 6072

Faculty of Dental Surgery
35/43 Lincoln's Inn Fields
London WC2A 3PN
Tel: 020 7312 6667

Royal College of Surgeons of England
35/43 Lincoln's Inn Fields
London WC2A 3PN
Tel: 020 7405 3474

Royal College of Surgeons in Ireland
123 St Stephen's Green
Dublin 2
Ireland
Tel: +35 31 402 2232

Faculty of Occupational Medicine
6 St Andrew's Place
Regent's Park
London NW1 4LB
Tel: 020 7317 5890

Royal College of Surgeons of Edinburgh
18 Nicolson Street
Edinburgh EH8
Tel: 0131 527 1600

Royal College of Nursing
20 Cavendish Square
London W1G 0RN
Tel: 020 7409 3333
www.rcn.org.uk/home/home.html

 **Think
Box**

I'm not sure if I would class the RCN as a Royal College or a trade union. A few years ago some nurse activists hijacked their annual conference and pushed through a vote to dump their 'no-strike' clause. It was a tense time for mainstream members. Now the CEO of the RCN is an American. Apparently there was no UK nurse up to the job. Don't believe it!

PRIMARY CARE ORGANISATIONS

 OK, listen up, this is important. You're going to have to read this bit! No shortcuts.

In April 2002, the reorganisation of the planning and commissioning system in the UK meant that the existing Health Authorities got dumped and the task of planning healthcare became the job of the Primary Care Trusts (PCTs) and Care Trusts.

There are 302 PCTs in England and two Care Trusts. I'd better add that three of them, Heart of Birmingham, Lincolnshire South West and Sunderland, are listed as Teaching PCTs – they get cross if you leave that bit out. Quite right too!

Details of all the PCTs can be found at:

• www.nhs.uk/localnhsservices/list_orgs.asp?ot=5__

NHS anoraks might like to know: www.doh.gov.uk/codes/datafiles.htm allows the codes and address of 302 PCTs to be downloaded. Useful if you're in the business of mailing for new customers and will save you money.

PCTs are responsible for spending over 70% of the healthcare budget. That figure is set to rise. The Government wants PCTs to run the whole show.

Over the next three years they will receive a revenue allocation of £148 billion. Allocations are made directly to the 304 Primary Care Trusts in England. An important change is that the allocations are for three years. This means PCTs can plan service over a longer period.

Good idea! Long overdue.

UNIVERSITY OF THE NHS

☹ Oh dear. Another initiative . . .

- www.nhsu.nhs.uk/

Most of the universities seem to be moaning they don't have enough money and the NHS is starting up its own. Do we need another uni? The NHS one claims it will be the largest uni in the world. Ho, hum . . .

It does have a rather entertaining turn of phrase:

> The NHS University will work with the one million staff in the NHS. It will be both a physical and virtual institution – using electronic and distance learning – the best of a 'bricks and clicks' approach, offering courses and training for every member of the NHS team whether they are nurses, doctors, therapists or cleaners.

. . . Bricks and clicks! I love it. Well done!

- The NHS University will help every member of NHS staff to reach their full potential – whether that is gaining NVQ qualifications for the first time to begin a career in nursing or training to undertake procedures previously done only by doctors.
- Everyone in the NHS will begin their career with the NHS University, through induction courses and direct training.
- The NHS University will deliver training in areas common to all health professionals from consultants to support workers, such as communication skills, ethics and assessment skills.
- Joint training between different health professionals, sharing their skills and experience and learning from each other will be a fundamental part of the NHS University curriculum.

Professor Robert Fryer has been appointed as chief executive designate for the NHS University and he's been busy sorting out a Memorandum of Understanding between the Department of Health and Universities UK over the development of the NHS University.

Well, it seems like a big old job to me. What happened to training departments? Do staff want these 'training opportunities', or do they want to come to work, do a job and go home to their families? I don't know.

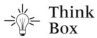
Think Box

I expect someone has done some in-depth market research amongst NHS staff to assess the uptake of all this and someone has done a feasibility study? I can't find one. If you know where it is, drop me an email at roylilley@compuserve.com.

Find the Uni at:

NHSU
Room 301a
Skipton House
80 London Road
London SE1 6LH

You can tell them what you think at yourviews@nhsu.nhs.uk. Or call them on 0800 555 550.

ENDNOTE

☺ OK, before you write to me, I expect I've left some organisations out. When I wrote this book I just scribbled out a list of outfits I thought were important, significant or worth including simply because they were so irrelevant to making sure granny got a new hip when she wanted one, I'd draw attention to them.

I've also included organisations that I wanted to pat on the back or have a dig at!

If you are in the book and are outraged, ask yourself, why? If you are not in the book, ask yourself, why?

Either way you can email me at roylilley@compuserve.com and give me a blast. When the next edition is being prepared I'll try and accommodate you!

INDEX

INDEX

staff *see* workforce strategy
star ratings 3, 5, 7, 10, 15
Stationery Office 72
StHAs *see* Strategic Health Authorities
strategic communications ('spin') 17, 23,
    32, 92
Strategic Health Authorities (StHAs) 28, 51,
    52, 53–4, 77
Structural Change in the NHS 68
super-trusts 61
supplies, NHS 25, 71–4
Supporting Doctors, Protecting Patients 45
SureStart 19

targets *see* performance management; star
    ratings
taxation 36, 58, 68
Teaching PCTs 97
technology *see* information technology
telephone health advice 47–9, 50
Thatcher, Margaret 4, 8, 51
Tory party 4, 8, 51
training, NHS 24, 28, 98
Trust Implementation Plans 66
Trusts *see* acute trusts; Care Trusts; NHS
    Trusts; Primary Care Trusts

UK Central Council for Nursing, Midwifery
    and Health Visiting 81
Universities UK 98
University of the NHS (NHSU) 23, 28,
    98–9

vCJD (variant Creutzfeldt-Jacob Disease)
    19
Veterinary Products Committee 38
voluntary organisations 56, 66, 69, 93

waiting times 7, 26
Wales, NHS 15, 45, 68–70, 78
Walk-in Centres 30–1
web skills *see* information technology
Wesson, Jane 46
The White Paper: Putting Patients First 70
whole systems planning 54
winter services management 20, 22
Witham, Braintree & Halstead Care Trust
    12
workforce strategy, NHS 23, 24, 28–9, 98

Zanamivir (Relenza) 37